Joy Amidst Friedreich's Ataxia

Deo Gloria — To God Be the Glory!

Joy Amidst Friedreich's Ataxia

Deo Gloria — To God Be the Glory!

David A. Keimig

XULON PRESS

Xulon Press
2301 Lucien Way #415
Maitland, FL 32751
407.339.4217
www.xulonpress.com

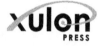

© 2023 by David A. Keimig

All rights reserved solely by the author. The author guarantees all contents are original and do not infringe upon the legal rights of any other person or work. No part of this book may be reproduced in any form without the permission of the author.

Due to the changing nature of the Internet, if there are any web addresses, links, or URLs included in this manuscript, these may have been altered and may no longer be accessible. The views and opinions shared in this book belong solely to the author and do not necessarily reflect those of the publisher. The publisher therefore disclaims responsibility for the views or opinions expressed within the work.

Unless otherwise indicated, Scripture quotations taken from the Holy Bible, New International Version (NIV). Copyright © 1973, 1978, 1984, 2011 by Biblica, Inc.™. Used by permission. All rights reserved.

Paperback ISBN-13: 978-1-66287-658-5
Ebook ISBN-13: 978-1-66287-659-2

To my parents, Mark and Carrie, for raising me in the ways of and guiding me to relationship with my Redeemer, as well as for many other reasons which I do not have the space to include here.

Acknowledgments

From the Joy Amidst Friedreich's Foundation, Inc.

Thank you David A. Keimig for being willing to share your story with the world. Your legacy will continue sharing the story of Christ for decades to come. Thank you to Xulon Press for assisting in the publication of this book.

From the Author

First off, thank you to my parents, Mark and Carrie, for establishing Joy Amidst Friedreich's Foundation, Inc. and thank you to the Foundation for funding the publication of my book. I am thankful and blessed to know that my story will result in charitable funds which can support other 501(c)(3) organizations. I am grateful to have had the opportunity to produce a written testimony, which I hope will encourage others and either strengthen faiths or play a role in leading others to a relationship with Jesus. With that, the Foundation and the author want to thank the various representatives with Xulon Press, for being so helpful in the various stages of book production.

Thank you to my loving family, my parents Mark and Carrie, my sister Jeanelle and husband Josh and my brother Daniel and wife Hope, and nieces and nephew who I love and are not yet at an age to realize their impact on my life. Thank you also to my Grandpa and Grandma Car, Vernon and Nona, who is no longer here. The relationships with both you and Grandma have been so dear and meaningful to me my entire life. You and Grandma were and are tremendous examples of what I hope to be as a Christian.

I am so thankful to be blessed with the rest of my family as well, my other grandparents, aunts and uncles, cousins, and beyond.

I would like to acknowledge my close friends, most of whom I have known since my childhood, Aaron, Matt Kok, Matt Klements, Tyler, and Geoff Scott "IB." I have learned that it is unusual for many people to have even one close friend from so many years ago and to still keep in touch with them. I thank each one of you and attest to your impact on my life and faith. We've had a lot of fun over the years and I am thankful, even though to a lesser degree, to still be a part of your lives

I would also like to add the full names of some of those people written about in the book including Adele Kroonenberg, Barbara Landhuis, Dee Dyk, Reba Bull, Chrysandra Brunson, Charity Seidler, Melissa Toerne, and Barbara Sipres. Obviously by including your names in my writing, my relationships with each of you are important to me! The same goes for those whose names are listed in the book but not written here. Thank you for your friendships and the years, some much longer than others, that you have remained a part of my life.

I would like to give a special thanks to Dave DeRidder, my friend, my former youth pastor, and in many ways a mentor. You have known me since I was dealing with my body falling apart throughout high school, and even since then, have been an encourager as I've faced difficulties. You are another whose Christian example is so great; I hope to emulate you as well. Know that you have made a huge impact on me!

Acknowledgments

Thank you to my friend Aaron's parents, Bruce and Carla Vandenberg. I have spent many hours around you since elementary school! You have been another set of people who have walked with and helped through my physical hardship. I am thankful for how our relationship has developed from me being a school friend of Aaron's, to getting to know you more and more, to traveling with you, keeping in touch and visiting with you currently, even when Aaron isn't around! You are another set of parents to me and I am thankful for you!

Thank you also to my friend Matt Klements' parents, Bob and Dottie Moore. I have also spent a lot of time around you since I met Matt through carpool. I was thankful to get to know you Bob, during the years doing that, especially when you would take us out to breakfast certain days before the start of school! You are yet another example of those who have lived with me through my trials. I am very thankful as well that we still keep in touch and visit with each other at times to maintain a relationship, apart from Matt (even though many times it does include Matt!) You both mean a lot to me, and you are another set of parents that I have.

There have been so many people in my life who impacted me and my faith along the way, whether it be other friends, classmates, teachers and professors, pastors, and many others from church. I could ponder and come up with so many names when I think about it!

I would like to thank all those who contributed to this book in some way. Thank you to my friend Cooper Pasque for both encouraging me to write and contributing to the book, my high school teacher René Meyer, and my pastors Mike James, and Timothy Milner. Thank you to Yvonne Howard MacKay for editing and contributing, for the hours you put in, and for the help you have given me beyond. I am thankful I have gotten to know you through this process! A large thank you to Bonnie Patterson for copyediting as well, and taking the time to do it while also teaching!

Lastly, I would like to acknowledge my dear and precious friend, Grace Soweidy. Grace and I first met in 2001 at my school, Denver Christian, where she was the custodian. Throughout high school, she would give me encouragement through Scripture or share jokes with me. She was always a very positive and joyful woman whenever anybody saw her. Though she was around 40 years older than me, we maintained a relationship after I had graduated; I would keep in touch with her and even though she eventually went on to Hawaii, we would make a point to visit each other whenever one or the other were nearby. Sadly, she died recently, but she was an amazing example of a loving and joyful Christian. My only sadness concerning this book is that she will not have the opportunity to read it.

Table of Contents

Foreword xv
Preface xix
Introduction xxiii

Chapter 1: Childhood Changes 1
Chapter 2: A Hard Blow 9
Chapter 3 Thankfully, an Unanswered Prayer 15
Chapter 4: Re-devotion 19
Truths I've Experienced: Blessing in Trials 23
Chapter 5: Something Suitable 29
Chapter 6: A Small Patch of Fat 35
Chapter 7: Graduating with a Walker 45
Chapter 8: Endings to New Beginnings 53
Truths I've Experienced: Strength in Weakness 55
Chapter 9: An Endearing Rule 63
Truths I've Experienced: Worry 69
Chapter 10: CCU, DC, & NY 75
Chapter 11: Unwelcomed News 83
Truths I've Experienced: On My Disability 101
Chapter 12: Capitol Calling 95
Truths I've Experienced: Relational Support 101
Chapter 13: Eyes Opened 105
Truths I've Experienced: Adversity 109
Chapter 14: Difficult Realities 117
Truths I've Experienced: Hope 131
Chapter 15: Voluntarily Visiting the Hospital 137
Chapter 16: Side Effects 141
Chapter 17: The New Year Begins with a Bang 145
Chapter 18: No More Fear 151

Truths I've Experienced: Joy 159
Chapter 19: Conclusion. 163

Afterword 175
References 179
Bibliography 181

The Good News

God created people to be in fellowship with Him (Genesis 1:26). After Adam and Eve sinned, humanity became separated from God (Genesis 3). Though over the centuries we have tried, no acts or deeds can be performed to make us right with God (Isaiah 64:6). Because of this, God sent his son Jesus to earth to fix our separation problem (John 3:16). Jesus was (and is) fully God and fully man. In God's great plan, Jesus lived a perfect life, was unjustly arrested, sentenced to death, and crucified—thus becoming the bearer of our sins (1 Corinthians 15: 3-4). Three days later, God raised Jesus from the dead, ultimately defeating sin and death (John 11: 25-26). Through Jesus—because of all He experienced, endured, and conquered—all of our sins—whether they are past, present, or future—can be forgiven by the grace that came from Christ's sacrifice. The only thing one must do to be forgiven is to choose to believe (Romans 5:1). Belief in Jesus as the one true God and His sacrifice brings forgiveness which leads to eternal life and glory with God (John 5:24). But unbelief in Jesus as Savior will lead to death and separation from God thereby leading to suffering for eternity (2 Thessalonians 1: 8-9, Acts 4:12, John 3:18). Jesus' sacrifice for our sin is the Good News brought and offered to us. The gift is free, and attaining it is simple (Romans 10: 9-10)!

Foreword

"I have told you these things, so that in me you may have peace. In this world you will have trouble. But take heart! I have overcome the world."

John 16:33

"For now we see only as a reflection as in a mirror; then we shall see face to face. Now I know in part; then I shall know fully, even as I am fully known."

I Corinthians 13:12

Friedreich's Ataxia—A condition that alters the nervous system and causes movement problems.

As a pre-teenager, David Keimig was an active, normal kid—busy in school activities, scouting, church, and many other pursuits. Little did Dave or his family know that his life was about to dramatically change. Dave had been diagnosed as having Friedreich's Ataxia. It was a difficult verdict for David to accept; his life would be so impacted. David continued his normal activities, but as time progressed, the ravages of this disease took their toll and he found it to be increasingly difficult to run, walk, and maintain his balance. It was determined, after many consultations, surgeries, and hospitalizations, that David's course of treatment would have to be to manage symptoms as they arose.

At this time, David has come to the realization that his disease cannot be cured by doctors, repaired by surgeries, or addressed by medicine. David was forced to turn to God, where his trust and hope were then and are now placed. David sees that life is not about his body or his personal comfort, but about being a witness for Christ by bringing others to Christ. David knows that God has blessed him and that this time of trial in his life is also a time of greatest blessing.

This isn't a new idea. Paul discussed such a paradox in Romans. "I consider that our present sufferings are not worth comparing with the glory that will be revealed in us." (8:18)."

As David is my grandson, I have seen him deal with the stages of impacts on his body as the Friedreich's Ataxia progressed. David went through initial stages of fear, grief, questioning, and finally acceptance of his condition. With the acceptance, David shows resilience and the determination that "this is not going to beat me". It became evident that he placed his life in God's hands. David has had peace and trust about where God leads him. David continued his involvement in Boy Scouts, achieving the rank of Eagle Scout. He entered Colorado Christian University and graduated with honors. I worked at the Colorado state capitol as a legislative aide. From his days in High School to the present, David has been part of a team to bring Bible studies to a nursing home. On the home front, David developed an interest in goats and developed a herd of more than three dozen of them. David found time to be a volunteer at Children's Hospital. In his spare time, David has travelled to every state in the United States, as well as to numerous countries overseas.

All that Dave has involved himself with has focused on bringing people to Christ. Never a complaint about his health,

David simply does not consider himself as disabled. His positive attitude and "can-do spirit" provide a great example of a Christian spirit. Undoubtedly, he has brought many people to Christ.

When all you have is God, you have all you need.

Vernon Ediger
(David's "Grandpa Car")

Preface

P.E. class and I had a love-hate relationship. I liked when we played games like Broomball, Zookeeper, or Dodgeball. Zookeeper was my favorite game. A group of kids in the middle of the gym were zookeepers who attempted to tag and "catch" the animals. The animals were the group of kids who ran to the other end of the gym, touched the stage, and ran back to the starting point—eluding contact with zookeepers. The animals were always chosen and I consistently was an alligator. I loved that game along with the other games, and was always excited when the teacher announced that our class time would consist of games or the giant parachute. Yet when we had to do exercises, I despised P.E.

I was not a lazy kid, but I hated running laps and doing wall-sits. We would often circle the school's carpeted gym, using a variety of modes of movement including: running, race-walking, skipping, and jumping. Wall-sits were primarily the punishment when somebody high-sticked during a game of Broomball.

For me, the most dreaded and hated times during the year in P. E. was the annual Presidential Fitness Assessment. (It may have only been once a year, but it sure seemed too often to me!) The assessment was made up of a series of exercises that each student was required to perform. Results were compared to other classmates, and also to a national standard. Students who did well earned a certificate signed by the president.

I could handle many of the required exercises. Pull-ups I could do. Running long-jump I could do. Relays I didn't like, but could do. The mile-long (600 yard) run, however, was the most wretched of all. My class walked to the field behind the school and was then told to run a number of laps within a certain time.

I don't remember how many laps it was, perhaps around five or six, but the total distance amounted to one mile. The field was large, and to me the distance, which I was given no choice about running, seemed laughably long. It turned out, I think, that I was never able to run the full distance because I took too long. Perhaps I did finish once; I do not remember.

Running long distances ... I despised it! However, there was one upside to the Presidential Fitness Testing. One of the exercises was a stretch, I forget what it was called. The student sat with their legs stretched in front of them on a board with some length markings at the end. The point was to lean over and stretch your fingertips as far past your toes as possible.

Now, I was very flexible; up through high school I was able to sit and bring both of my ankles behind my head. So, this stretch exercise I could do! I was good, and usually in the top numbers for this exercise. I never got a certificate though, as my stretching results combined with my other results were insufficient to get me a certificate. That was unfortunate, but I honestly could not have cared less.

Alas, I did not look forward to P.E. with eager expectation. I recall a particular day when I was in the sixth grade. When P.E. class finished, everyone cleaned up and started to leave for the next class. Mrs. Landhuis, the P.E. teacher, pulled me aside and told me someone wanted to see me briefly.

Mrs. Landhuis and I went onto the stage—the open area behind the curtains. There stood a woman whom I had never seen. She asked if I would do some short exercises. Being compliant, I did. The one I most vividly remember involved my running back and forth in a straight line, touching tape at the ends. I think she even had me doing something where I'd touch her finger and then my nose, with my index finger, as quickly and accurately as I could. About ten minutes later when I finished, the woman thanked me, and Mrs. Landhuis sent me on my way to my next class. I remember thinking, *Who in the world was that lady, and what was that all about?*

Introduction

Prior to sharing more about myself, I must first give what I call my "disclaimer" before I go any further; I write this book and give this testimony solely for the glory of God. My intention is not to encourage the reader to think highly of me, nor for me to elevate myself or my status at all. This testimony is not for the glorification of myself, but of God—without whom my life would be trivial.

My name is David Alan Keimig. Keimig is pronounced with a silent "e" and a long "i," but most people have no idea how to pronounce this great German name. The most common errors people make when attempting to say Keimig are by pronouncing it "Keemig," "Keimick," "Keiming," or "Kaemig." I hope David is not too difficult to sound out.

At the time of this writing, I am in my younger 30's, and a native Coloradan. I have lived most of my life in suburban Aurora, but currently reside on the plains outside of a growing small town named Bennett, a little east of Denver. My family is comprised of my parents Mark and Carrie, me—their eldest, my sister Jeanelle, and my brother Daniel. My siblings and I each have two years between us. My two in-laws are Josh and Hope, and I am greatly blessed to be an uncle six times over, to Grace, Julia, Caleb, Nora, Finley, and Piper. I have a number of aunts, uncles, and cousins, and grew up with both sets of grandparents nearby. As a child I designated my grandparents by the vehicles they owned, so the Edigers are Grandma and Grandpa Car, and the Keimigs are Grandma and Grandpa Jeep.

I live with my parents, not out of slothfulness, but because of my circumstances. For the same reason, I am single as well.

As I hope you surmise, it sounds like I'm a pretty regular guy, right? Well, I am. I don't have a famous name. I've never done anything spectacular. And unless you're a friend or family member, you've never heard of this David with a last name you don't know how to say.

I'll show you how average and, perhaps, quirky, I am. For fun I like to target-shoot, read, watch movies or television, play video games, create designs for my 3D printer, and assemble plastic model kits. I like listening to music, preferring Classical, John Philip Sousa marches, and hymns/Gospel over modern music because much modern music is rubbish. I love my country, and I like baseball, NASCAR, trains, and the Olympics. I enjoy symphonies, musicals, and operas (so hey, I'd say I'm cultured). I love being outside, traveling, and learning. I also simply love to do—to try new things, to participate, and to have fun.

So whoop-dee-do, yes? If I'm so average in many ways, why should you bother reading a book about my life; it's probably not terribly exciting, eh?

Well, that's a brief glimpse into my interests, but through my short three decades of life, my body has changed greatly, and will continue to do so. My relationship with Christ—though I've had it since a young age—has taken on deeper meaning because of the difficulties I constantly face every day. Because of my obvious outward-trials, I've been renewed inwardly and gained unique insights on life and the Lord's truly active role in it.

Introduction

I wrote this book about my life, where I've come from, what I've been through, and where I am now. Interspersed throughout this book I have inserted what I have called "Truths I've Experienced." I feel these truths have been shown to me through living each day with a trial, and through which I hope to proclaim the lessons I have learned. I am not a theologian or biblical scholar, so these various points in the chapters ahead are what I live by to the best of my ability according to the understanding I have. These ideas are my original thoughts; they back the expression of conclusions I have come to as I have walked by faith through my personal trials. These chapters are what I most love to think about, and sharing those ideas gives me joy. God's glory is, at many times, shown through instances in which it seems unlikely that joy could come. I hope and pray that these ideas will be a witness and encouragement as you read them.

This book is written as an encouragement and as a witness—not to how great I, as a mere person, am. Rather, it is written to God's glory, for the wonder of how He has been faithful to me, and for the truth that what He has done is sufficient for you—if your faith is in Him. The following are my experiences and what I believe the Lord has taught me through what I've faced.

Chapter 1

Childhood Changes

From the time of my first breath, the Lord has blessed me tremendously. I was born to loving parents who, over the years, provided a stable household with its foundation built upon Christ. I was born an apparently-healthy child, without illness or disability. I grew to be a chubby and very cute baby—so I am told!

When Jeanelle and Daniel arrived two and four years later, life became much more fun. We all loved to play together. Since, thankfully, we didn't have video games until I was about ten, we spent much of the time playing outside and using our imaginations. Actually, my dad did have an Atari, and Nell won a Sega at age two, but these were rarely used. We rode our bikes, chased our chickens, swam with each other in the stock tank, or played in the dirt pile. We had fun together—even though we irritated each other every now and then.

Yet my parents, themselves each one of five kids, say my siblings and I were odd. We'd have tiffs and arguments here and there, but never got into fights or huge arguments, while my parents' and other families I've observed could spar intensely. The relationships between Nell, Dan and me were certainly not perfect, but were pretty amicable and out of the ordinary.

From since I can remember, I was raised going to church and learning about the Bible and Jesus' sacrifice for mankind.

My brother and I wore our dapper little suits to church, and Jeanelle her fancy little dresses. We went to Sunday School, sang in the children's choir, and grew up with three grandparents along with several other relatives attending the same church.

In addition to what I learned at church, my parents raised me in a Christian manner at home. They led me in God's truth and taught me in His ways. I loved Sunday School songs so much. I often went outside to the swing set in the mornings and belted out my favorites—apparently to the delight of my mom and the neighbors.

I arrived quickly and unexpectedly into my parents' new marriage. My mom, a third-grade teacher, became a stay-at-home mom. When my mom was pregnant with my sister, my parents found an affordable house in a less desirable part of the city. The part of town in which we lived had a poor public education school system, and my parents wanted their children in a private educational setting, where their values would be taught.

Affording a private education would present some challenges. My family wasn't poor, but we didn't have a great amount of money. My dad was a concrete laborer at a small concrete foundation company, and also fueled airplanes at Stapleton Airport. Dad talked with his boss at the concrete company about his desire to provide a private education for his children. His boss suggested my parents look at Denver Christian.

As the years went on, the time for me to start kindergarten came. God greatly blessed me by placing me in a situation through which I would be amazingly blessed even for many years into my future.

Denver Christian is a small, private school which was located in Denver (now Lakewood), backed by the very Dutch, Christian Reformed Church. Mom and Dad, unsure of how they would pay for a private education, put their trust in God and enrolled me. My siblings and I each attended Denver Christian from kindergarten through high school. Only later did we learn that our parents routinely received anonymous gifts of money for tuition. Those anonymous gifts gave them the help and provision needed to keep us enrolled. Neither my parents nor I knew the impact this school would have on my life.

When I turned five, I went to kindergarten at Van Dellen—one of Denver Christian's small elementary schools. I was from Aurora, a good half-an-hour away, so I didn't know anyone at this school. But that soon changed. I was in Mrs. Ten Broek's morning kindergarten class, and while I made friends, it wasn't until both kindergarten classes took a field trip to a dairy farm together that I made my best friends. Somehow, three boys—Matt Kok, Aaron Vandenberg, and myself—from different classes got together and hit it off. I have an enduring friendship with both Matt and Aaron even today.

Elementary school was great. Although my closest friends and I were usually in different classes, I did get to see them many times either in passing or at recess. I loved all my teachers and made sure to frequently hug them. I even made sure to give the secretary, Mrs. Kroonenberg, a hug each day before I left!

Each time I entered the school, it had the same distinct smell. As the years went on, I always associated that smell with my school. It was a nice, sweet scent that hit the nose each time I entered, and although I didn't know where it came from, I always knew I was in the right place because of it. Little did I know that years later, and quite accidentally, I would discover that the scent came from a perfume worn by Mrs. Kroonenberg!

Besides the usual squabbles and disagreements elementary schoolers have with each other, I never had any large problems with anyone. In second grade, I was even asked (through a note) by a girl if I would like to be her fiancé. I took that note home and asked my mom, "What is a fee-ance?" Unbeknownst to me, this girl *really* liked me and wanted to be engaged to me—in second grade! Wow! After learning that, I asked, "What does engaged mean?" However, after I learned what fiancé and engaged meant, I wanted nothing to do with it!

While I was in the fourth grade, I also developed a close friendship with Matt Klements. He was my sister's age—a second-grader. This developed largely because our families carpooled. While at Van Dellen, I developed many relationships, both with fellow students and faculty. The community and environment were terrific, and the Christian setting reinforced what I had learned and continued to learn at home and in church. Elementary school was also the time when my friend Aaron encouraged me to join Cub Scouts. Scouts opened up another avenue for me to get to know people and provided me with many fun adventures as well.

Well, now is the time that we catch up from the beginning of the book. As I was about to complete elementary school—which, in Colorado at the time, ended with sixth grade—and when middle school was on the horizon, I had the strange experience in my sixth grade P.E. class (as I described before). Life was great, life was normal, and in my sixth-grade mind I had no difficulties to face except for P.E. and math class. P.E. may have been a love-hate relationship, but math was one of pure spite. To this day I still hate math. I'm still not very good at it, but I don't mind the elementary basics of addition, subtraction, simple multiplication, and simple division. I decided long ago that when I get married, I hope it is to somebody who is good—or at least decent—at math to counter me when it comes to bills and taxes. Anyway, life was good, so again, what was this encounter with the lady who asked me to run lines and touch my nose all about?

Shortly after that experience, I learned that that my parents were becoming concerned about my coordination. At the time, I did not fully understand what my coordination did for me, so I wasn't really worried about it. I was a young sixth-grader; I could run, play sports, and do whatever I wanted. In my mind, there was no reason to think it would ever be otherwise. Not long after this however, the fun of frequently visiting doctors ensued.

My family was well acquainted with doctors, however. By the age of nine, I had already had three eye surgeries, and when my brother was nine, he had already had nine eye surgeries and had been to the hospital a number of times for asthma-related issues. My sister was the lucky one; she didn't have any physical maladies that needed correcting.

In my life I'd already learned the joys of visiting the doctor: the long wait times, the boring magazines for people to read in the waiting room, and the un-inviting sterile smell of the office. Little did I know, this joy in my life would become greatly multiplied. It was not until I started seeing more doctors that I started to feel that something was off.

The results of the exercises I had done for the woman after P.E. class showed that my coordination was not normal for my age. My parents took me to see doctors of all kinds. It started with my general physician, who then worked with my parents to find other specialists who may be able to diagnose why my coordination had worsened. I remember going to see a neurologist, and I had no idea why I would need to see one of those.

I remember learning that a neurologist deals with brain and nerve issues, but at that age, this seemed like a stretch.

It wasn't until going to see another doctor that a few things were clarified. I vividly remember a small doctor's office in the middle of Aurora. My mom and I were there to see yet another doctor. I don't even remember what kind of doctor he was, but I do recall the experience.

We went back to a small office and I'm sure I did the usual dog-and-pony show demonstrating my coordination through various exercises until the doctor left, probably to consult or to research. After a wait, the doctor came back, and told us his opinion. This doctor had poor bedside manner, and I experienced him as terribly insensitive and unsympathetic. My mother was very upset with the way this doctor laid out this information to me.

He explained, with me sitting right there, that I could potentially have an incurable degenerative disorder (meaning it would continually worsen over time) called Friedreich's Ataxia. He stated that if this was an accurate diagnosis, it would explain why my coordination had worsened. He went on to say that if I had this disorder, I eventually may not be able to walk or to drive, I may end up with heart and other issues, and there is no cure. This unexpected news really freaked me out! The only way to test this doctor's theory would be for me to get a blood test, as the disorder is genetic.

I remember this as having been an awful day. My mom and I had gone to a doctor—who having no bedside manner—delivered, in the least tactful way possible, this awful news to a child. All of this information was left to float around in my mind. This was a very scary time for me as a young kid. Here I had a good body—I could walk, run, jump, go anywhere I wanted… Yet now I was faced with the prospect of thinking that as I grew older, I may lose all of that. I had to comprehend that over time, my body may fall apart, and that my future may not include many of the things that, until this very moment, I had assumed it would.

As you can guess, this news was hard not only on me, but on my family as well. I know now that my parents had a much harder time reconciling this than I did. Here we had a great family—three healthy kids, a stable home, and a strong marriage between my parents. Now it seemed that their oldest child may have a hard road ahead of him. It was hard news on my brother and sister as well. Of course, nothing had happened yet, but the fears of what the future may hold scared all of us.

I remember a time where all of us sat out on our front steps to talk about what might happen if it was found that I had this disorder. My parents explained what the disorder was, and we wondered why God may have been allowing this. We talked about what this disorder could mean for the future. The discussion brought many tears from everybody, as well brought renewed prayers and trust in the Lord for whatever the future would hold.

My sixth-grade year came and went. I had seen so many doctors that I hated the thought of visiting one more. A new school year started—my first year in middle school, seventh grade……

Chapter 2

A Hard Blow

Starting middle school was exciting. All of my good friends were still at school, and now we were even closer together in the small space of Denver Christian Middle School. I had new teachers, new classes, and a bit more freedom to roam about between them.

I loved certain classes such as a Geography and U.S. History, but absolutely hated others like pre-Algebra. Near the beginning of my first semester of middle school, my parents decided to have my blood tested to discover if I had Friedreich's Ataxia. This was another trying time in my life.

Depending on the results of the blood test, I either had or didn't have that awful disorder, and prospects for my future seemed at stake. The test results took about a month (if I remember correctly), so I had plenty of time to digest my thoughts concerning whether I had Friedreich's Ataxia or not.

Each day, the four homerooms in my middle school had devotionals before class started. And each day at this time, I was in my math class with Mrs. Woudstra. And each morning I had a big prayer request: I asked for prayer regarding the blood test I had taken, that God would bless the result, and that the test would come back negative—showing that I didn't have the disorder. That was prayed and it remained a prayer until the results arrived.

My relationship with, and reliance on God grew during this period. The time I spent traveling to see doctors to get opinions helped me to pray more frequently, and it further increased my trust in God. I prayed constantly for a negative result, and I know I'm not the only one who did.

My parents and siblings were in prayer, as were extended family and many friends. I didn't know whether or not my prayers would be answered in the way I and others desired, but there was no doubt in my mind that the Lord had the ability to alter the situation. Those around me also had this mind-set, and what encouragement that gave me!

Well, one day the results came back. I honestly do not even remember how or when I heard the news. However, the outcome was clear: My genes matched up. I had Friedreich's Ataxia. This was sobering news and let me further explain why.

Friedreich's Ataxia is named after a German doctor who described its symptoms in the 1860's. The word "ataxia" has to do with one's nerves and involuntary muscle movements. Friedreich's Ataxia tends to show up in people during their elementary to teenage years. Less often, its symptoms can appear in one's 20's or 30's also. As for me, at age 11, I was within the normal range for it to be discovered.

This genetic, neuromuscular disorder can be indicated through symptoms of lack of coordination, an irregular gait, or loss of sensation in the lower extremities. I only showed the first. The mutated gene is recessive, meaning that the disorder can skip generations in a family, and both parents must be carriers of the gene for a child to inherit it. Symptoms over one's lifetime include those characteristics mentioned above. Additionally, there may be a loss of balance, increased frequency of falling, the loss of the ability to walk, scoliosis (curvature of the spine), slurred speech, problems with eyesight and/or hearing, highly-arched feet, diabetes, increased fatigue, difficulty with swallowing, and a host of heart problems.

Each person who has Friedreich's Ataxia shows different symptoms, and the severity of symptoms varies widely among those who have the disorder. Being a degenerative disorder, symptoms of Friedreich's Ataxia will progressively worsen over time when they appear. Once an ability is lost, it cannot be regained. This news absolutely scared me, but here was the kicker: there is no cure for Friedreich's Ataxia. To clarify, my brief explanation of Friedreich's Ataxia is accurate, but not fully exhaustive.

The only hopeful news relating to this diagnosis is that as I grow older, my body may get to a point at which the symptoms plateau. Additionally, it is possible that I won't develop each of these symptoms. I was able to find these few positives hidden in the onslaught of this diagnosis.

You may read the following and think I am a fool. Or you may read it and think that I have a tiny bit of wisdom. My knowledge of Friedreich's includes what my doctors have told me, what I have personally experienced, and what I have learned from the small amount I have read about it.

Having a specific disorder, I do want to be overly-informed on the disorder—what the symptoms are, and what future symptoms may occur. However, I have chosen to remain somewhat ignorant of all of the details and potential future symptoms. Why? I believe that while it is important to know what I have, it is more important that I live my life and deal with things as they come, as opposed to knowing all of the potential problems and living in fear and anxiety of whether or not more difficulty may come into my life. I have offered a basic explanation of Friedreich's and its symptoms, and if you want to know all the nitty-gritty about it, I invite you to look it up yourself. As for me, I don't feel the need.

Even at the time of the diagnosis, my body still wasn't showing many signs of being much different from the body of anyone else I knew. After learning (from that awful, tactless doctor), when I was all of 11 years of age, what Friedreich's Ataxia is, I and those around me fervently prayed that I would be spared from this disorder. But then I got the news that I definitely have this disorder, and suddenly my future terrified me.

I realized that I would watch what looked like my healthy body fall apart over time. I considered that among other things, I may lose my ability to walk. I understood that I would probably see my life go from being independent to having to rely on others to help me with very basic things in my everyday life. And I understood that there was absolutely nothing anybody could do about it. I'm sure that this prospect is daunting for anybody at any age, but being so young and healthy, this took much of the wind of hope for my future out of my sails.

I can say that the Lord had shaped me in my young life, to where I didn't take the news out on Him. This shaping was not by my own doing, nor by my own strength. I don't know why, but I did not feel the need to blame God for this misfortune. It was a hard blow, but I figured that rather than being mad at God, putting my trust in Him and seeking His help as my body deteriorated in the future was more important. I didn't, and still don't, know why God allowed *me* to be born with this disorder.

I did not believe (and still don't believe) that God *gave* me such an awful thing. I do believe that He allowed it as He allowed Satan to bring trouble upon Job. My diagnosis was (and still is) much harder for my parents to deal with than it is for me.

A Hard Blow

Not being a parent, I cannot completely empathize with bearing the knowledge that your child will lose much of what you hoped they would have in their future, but I know it shook their lives and tested their faith. This news rippled in my small community. From my grandparents, aunts and uncles, friends, teachers, and people at church; it was hard for all to accept. The only thing we could do was watch and see what God had planned for my future.

I soon learned that despite the mystery having finally been dispelled by the diagnosis, the continuation of seeing an endless line of doctors did not dampen. Friedreich's is a rare disorder, so doctors and medical school students alike were intrigued to see and to study someone with what I have.

I quickly started visiting the Muscular Dystrophy Association Muscle Clinic at Colorado Children's Hospital, a place I was becoming uncomfortably familiar with. The Muscle Clinic served children with various forms of muscular dystrophy whom they monitored, examined, and suggested either treatment or exercises. Friedreich's is not a form of muscular dystrophy, but since those with Friedreich's exhibit similar symptoms, I was able to be seen at the MDA Muscle Clinic.

Many of the staff were very knowledgeable about my situation. Everything about this environment and about the disorder itself was new to me, and seeing the other patients and their bodies, I felt out of place. Little did I know that in the coming years I would fit right in.

Chapter 3

Thankfully, an Unanswered Prayer

After being diagnosed in early seventh grade, the rest of the school year went well. I can't say that this was reflected in my grades, but I enjoyed school. Now school was out and the summer was about to begin. As I have said, I still visited the medical community frequently after my diagnosis. During the summer, the next big change in my life began to gin up.

As I mentioned in the description of Friedreich's, a potential symptom is scoliosis. I'm no brainiac doctor, but here's a layman's description of it. Scoliosis is when one's spine begins to bend or curve in the torso. Not only can scoliosis ruin one's posture, but it is also dangerous in that, if it continues to curve unchecked, it can present a danger to the organs as the vertebrae may puncture them.

Sometime during that summer, one of my doctors wanted me to have an x-ray taken just to see whether or not I had scoliosis. This was another typically fun doctor's appointment as well. Upon looking at the x-ray results, I was informed that my spine was indeed curving, and that having caught it, the doctor deemed it necessary that I have a spinal fusion surgery to prevent further curvature.

Spinal fusion surgery is what it sounds like. Surgeons put titanium rods up against the spine, screw them into the bone, and make a box-like structure, thus, fusing the bones together and preventing any further movement of the spine.

As you see, this was another day of great news, but it did get better. The good news was that I did not need the surgery urgently—as in I did not need the surgery that summer. But the bad news was that I would probably need it during the next school year. Within a year, I had two large burdens placed upon me, but little did I know how life-changing this surgery would be.

I began eighth grade: my second year of middle school. I was excited about school because this was the final year of middle school and, while portions of it were fun, I was ready to get into high school. Even though I was looking forward to high school, this did not diminish the pleasure I had in seeing so many familiar faces of friends and teachers.

With this new year, came a new prayer. Rather than prayer requests about a diagnosis, the new request was for prevention of the necessity for spinal fusion surgery. Again, many people in my life were praying not only for my healing from the disorder, but also for the healing of my back so that I would not have to go through this invasive surgery.

Within my family, we talked and prayed constantly about the surgery and about God being sovereign and His power to do all things. While we prayed and hoped that the surgery would not be necessary, we also knew of, and prayed for, the Lord's blessing on whatever may happen, surgery or not. As the surgery date, January 9, 2001, loomed ever closer, many around me gave great encouragement and love.

At the end of December, a few weeks prior to my surgery date, I had to go to the hospital and meet someone who would give me the pre-operation talk. They told me about the procedure, and that not the entire length of my spine needed to be fused, only from just under my neck to the lower part of my back.

I was told that when I woke up after surgery, I'd have an IV, something on my finger (which I now know is called a Pulse Ox), potentially a tube down my throat to provide air for my lungs … and a catheter. I had never heard of a catheter before, and after learning what it was, that device made me anxious! I really did not want that thing. (Not to be explicit, but this is basically a small tube that is inserted into the bladder so that it can be automatically drained while the patient is in surgery, bed, or otherwise unable to physically urinate; I'll leave it up to you to guess where the tube goes!)

I was also told about the recovery time in and out of the hospital. The average in-hospital recovery time for someone who has had spinal fusion surgery was nine days. I thought, O*ver my dead body!* The recovery time after leaving the hospital was a number of months—six I believe. I left the pre-op appointment feeling even more nervous about the procedure.

The time leading up to the surgery was speeding by, and my family and I hoped healing would come and that I wouldn't have to undergo a spinal fusion. While school was out over Christmas break, we strengthened our reliance on God. I remember a specific conversation I had with my friend Aaron over the phone only days before the surgery.

In the course of our conversation, I specifically remember telling Aaron, whom I could not see before the surgery, "Keep praying for God's healing of my spine because I know that I can be in the hospital, lying on that table about ready to go unconscious, and God can choose to heal me then and there." Aaron promised he would continue to pray. Thankfully, the Lord didn't answer those prayers!

Chapter 4

Re-devotion

The day of the surgery—January 9, 2001—arrived. As instructed, I'd fasted the night before. Early that morning, my parents took me to the hospital. As you might expect, I was fairly jittery. Waiting with me before I was prepped for the surgery were my parents along with Grandpa and Grandma Car. Also present was an elder from my church. Before I went back to be prepped for surgery, I received the best encouragement I could have been given before this major event.

Everyone who was there took turns praying. My dad's prayer gave me great hope by reminding me that I had absolutely no control over what would take place. He prayed that God would protect me during the surgery and guide the surgeon's hands. The time soon came, and I went back to the preparation area with my dad.

The nurse had me put on a gown and instructed me to lie down on a gurney. She poked the IV in, and put a mask over my face. The anesthesiologist had me count to 10. I started, "One, two, three, four..." and the last thing I saw was my dad looking at me, and I was out.

The next thing I remember was briefly waking in a fog and seeing a large group of family members looking at me and congratulating me. I quickly fell back asleep. I woke up sometime later—a bit more alert—and was informed that the surgery had gone well. I was thankful for the success, however, having my back cut open and my spine shifted was fairly painful, despite the powerful painkillers I was given.

Initially, being in the hospital after the surgery turned out not to be all bad. Let me clarify: being *in* the hospital... I absolutely hated, but all the staff were a blessing and an encouragement to me. One thing that did not take me long to figure out as a middle school boy, was how much I appreciated the pretty nurses who attended to my needs. Even in my sometimes foggy, and always somewhat painful, state, I made a point to be courteous, cordial, and thankful to the nurses. It seemed that they quite enjoyed having me as a patient —appreciating my temperament and my attitude. Likewise, I quite valued the great care from them!

I was relieved that my stay in the hospital would not be a lonely one. To start with, at least one of my parents stayed with me day and night the whole time. Jeanelle and Daniel were often there after school in the afternoons. I frequently had visits from grandparents, aunts and uncles, and close friends as well.

Another terrific part of my hospital recovery was that nearly each afternoon, I had numerous visitors from my school. To my surprise, most of my teachers visited me in the hospital. Many of my other fellow students came to see me too—even classmates with whom I did not interact much. Each of these visitors strengthened me with their encouragement during my time in the hospital.

I vividly recall one visit from a teacher and about four other classmates. During the course of the visit, I felt the need to urinate very badly, but was unable to go. As I was enjoying the company, I didn't say anything until my guests left, because I didn't want to hasten their exit. When they were gone, I told my parents and they pushed the nurse "call" button.

A nurse came in and said "Oh! That means that it's time for the catheter to come out." As I knew how the catheter was inserted, I was wary of how it would be removed. As I type these words I still shudder at this recollection. In the most barbaric of ways, the nurse just yanked it out! That pain was worse than any of the other pain I remember from the surgery itself. I understand the catheter's usefulness, and I'm sure it is equally as unpleasant for a woman to have one, but for guys, it's an absolute torture device!

Apart from both the irritations and good situations and events during my hospital stay, my life changed in another way because of the need for this surgery. Now that I'd had the surgery, rather than praying about that, my focus was re-directed. I knew, that the recovery from the surgery was not going to be easy and that I needed help to get through it. After I became lucid—when the anesthesia wore off—I started praying intensely that the Lord would provide me strength to help me to carry on as well as give me motivation. I really didn't want to be in the hospital for nine days.

Trusting and relying on God, I was able to stay strong. When I had to do the seemingly-silly breathing and physical exercises I needed to complete in order to eventually leave the hospital, I did not give up despite pain and fatigue. I did not go through a time when I had a bad attitude or feared the pain and struggle of recovery. God showed His love to me and gave me encouragement and motivation through the generosity of the people He sent to me.

Through that week, the Lord showed me that I could rely on Him and the hope of salvation; not only to persevere through a difficult time, but also to serve Christ and show His love to others through tribulation. As I've shared before, I grew up as a Christian. In the Christian community, many people who have converted are able to tell you the exact day it happened. Well, I can't. I was raised in a Christian household, and after processing the message of Christ and what it meant for me, I prayed with my dad at a young age to accept Christ as my Savior. The best I can say is that I was seven I years old or under. I was baptized at a young age as well, but I don't remember specifically when that occurred either. Although I don't remember the dates or all the details, I do remember these experiences.

The experience of this surgery and the time I spent in the hospital matured my faith. Having seen and experienced firsthand God's truths playing out in my life, my faith developed. I took my faith on as my own and began to grow increasingly devoted to it.

There is a time in each person's life, Christian or unbeliever when one must make a decision to dedicate one's life to one's beliefs. For the one who has heard the Good News, this is the moment in which one ultimately accepts or rejects Jesus. That moment certainly differs in each person's life. But that also doesn't mean that if you become a Christian as a child, your faith isn't sincere.

I accepted Christ as a child, and my faith was sincere; the time simply came for me to decide whether I, in further maturity, wanted to remain in Christ and more deeply devote my life to Him. With my life circumstances, that wasn't a hard decision for me. Others might respond differently because of their situation and decide not to believe in God. I understand this and hope that my testimony might persuade readers in that mind frame to reconsider.

Truths I've Experienced

Blessing in Trials

> And we know that in all things God works for the good of those who love him, who have been called according to his purpose.
>
> Romans 8:28

Persevering through all the trials I have faced, and continue to face, in my life, my physical state being the most predominant, the hope I have from being a Christian is extremely important to my outlook on life. As you continue to read, you'll observe that hope is a continual theme in my life.

In the book of Romans, we're given a distinct promise of hope from the Bible. It is found in Romans 8:28. If we love God and devote our lives to serving Him, God will use every happening in our lives to our benefit, increasing His glory through us for others to see Him!

This obviously means that the blessings and good times in our lives will be for good. It also means that the bad times in our lives—the difficulties, weaknesses, hardship, insults, and persecution—will also be used for good. Our decisions (whether good or bad), and our hardships, will be used by God to develop our character, to mold us, and to strengthen us in the faith. The Lord is omnipotent: He is all-powerful, and His promise is not that the good will bless us and the bad will harm us, but that both the good and the bad in life will be used to bring about His Kingdom and also to make the individual better and stronger.

Even at my young age at the time of my diagnosis, I understood that, as I had no control over my circumstances, I could only trust in God for my future. Romans 8:28 is a verse in which the meaning is very clear to me. Other Christians who have sought God's help through a trial in their lives also have a strong understanding of this promise. This verse may be easy to read over, and simply think, *that's nice*, and move on. Until one is in the midst of a trial, or especially coming out of a trial, the words may not permeate as well.

Why would all, or any, of the pitfalls of life be to a believer's benefit? Sure, the unbeliever who faces a trial may come out of it feeling stronger, but ultimately, what is the end goal? What is the purpose? I (and I'm certainly not alone) can proclaim that as a Christian, my greatest blessings have not come in times of joy, happiness, abundance, or material blessings, but instead in times of trial and hardship. Frankly, the most blessed seasons in my life have been the worst!

Allow me to try to explain this. In the hard times of my life, I could not then, and I cannot now rely on my own strength. I turn to God and to His Word—not only to give me the hope to persevere through the difficult time, but also because He has the power to take away whatever I face. If we turn to God, times of difficulty in our lives will strengthen our relationship with, increase our trust in, and develop our reliance on Him.

In dark times God's presence seems to strengthen. We feel His encouragement so much more when we truly need Him than we do when our lives are going "our way". During these easy times of selfishness and obliviousness, our focus tends to wander from God, and we lose sight of His daily work in our lives. In trials, we can live as we should, putting our faith and trust in God—in the forefront of our minds and hearts—and discover His encouragement and love in our daily lives no matter what we face.

Yet Christians who see that the greatest blessings in life come out of trials certainly do not look forward to trials yet to come. Times of trial yield blessings, but the trials are undeniably horrible when one is in the midst of such a storm. Often, it takes a prolonged period after the trial has ended for the afflicted to see the good in it.

Many times, God may choose not to show us the good that came from a certain time in our lives. I look back to the time in college when I had a fit of anxiety for a month or so. I have no idea how God was using that in my life, because when the anxiety went away, I didn't (and still don't) see any betterment in myself from having gone through that. But even though I do not see it, believing that God's promise in Romans 8:28 is true, I have the confidence that in some way God used that time in my life for good—mine or someone else's. Other times, it is very clear to me what the benefit of a trial may be.

I have a surprising thought that will likely seem completely non-sensical and perhaps outright ludicrous, but hear me out. As I pray, I often think about the changes in my body since I started to be affected by Friedreich's Ataxia. I sometimes dwell on my disorder and reflect on how—since it is genetic—doctors cannot fix it, medicine cannot heal it, and surgery cannot repair it. Nothing in this world can take it away. This brings me great joy!

In spite of the fact that there is no human cure for Friedreich's Ataxia, I have a relationship with the Almighty Lord. He has the power to touch me and bring the miracle of healing! With no current cure, the world cannot heal my body, but my God can. In a way, I have been fortunate because I've been forced to trust in God in this area. I cannot rely on medicine, doctors and surgeons, technology, or procedures, so my trust and hope truly is in the Lord.

What a tremendous, joyful feeling it is to have trust and hope in only Christ. I am imperfect, so I don't always put as much trust in God as I should, but it is great to know that I do not have to trust in the world, but rather rely on faith and on the power of God.

I pray, and have prayed, many times that He would heal my body. I know that this would be a very simple deed for the Lord. I pray for that, and if I'm healed, there will be joyous celebration; if I'm not, there will still be joy in my life. Whether my body is ever healed or never healed in this lifetime is not important. I've yearned for and desired healing for years, and will continue to, but my life is not about my body or my comfort; it's about leading people to Christ and being a witness by sharing how God has worked in my life.

Times of trial are mostly horrible times in our lives. During such times we can experience despair, anger, and hopelessness. I have been living with a daily trial for 21 years now, and it still stinks!

I still find times where I revert to pitiful feelings about my situation. But those feelings come from the Enemy, and it is best not to be overwhelmed with them. Those who turn to God will be bestowed with blessings. This is the promise to each person who believes. As we live loving God, we will be blessed through the times of happiness in our lives, but we will be more deeply enriched through the difficulties we face. God loves us with such unfathomable love; He uses not only our happiness and joy, but also, our sadness, doubt, anger, hopelessness, despair and screw ups, for our good.

Chapter 5

Something Suitable

High school was a wonderful time in my life. When I think back, the positives far outweigh the negatives. The school at the time averaged about 350 students, so my class was not very big. By my frame of reference, that was large, but compared to public schools it was very small. I didn't have much trouble adapting to high school. My friends were in my classes, and I got to see them frequently. I didn't have trouble with other kids. I liked getting to know new teachers and having a greater variety of, and more demanding, classes. (However, I liked challenges only in certain subjects. Those that I didn't want challenges in, I found challenging enough as they were!)

Having completed eighth grade in May of the same calendar year as my spinal fusion, my recovery from that surgery was pretty much complete by the time I began high school. At this point in time— two years since my diagnosis and seven months since my surgery—I had not seen many of the symptoms of Friedreich's Ataxia.

Early in my freshman year, however, the first symptom I noticed began to manifest. Walking the hallways of my high school, books in hand, I felt myself teeter slightly. I could walk in the middle of an open corridor but suddenly lose my balance a bit and shift to one side. At the time it seemed odd as I'd never had that happen before, but I still didn't put too much credence into it. I knew I could not walk in a straight line, for even as a child when I attempted to walk on the balance beams in parks, I was unable to do so. However, at my regular evaluations at the Muscle Clinic, I was warned that poor balance was an early sign of degeneration from my disorder.

Well, time went on and life was good. Though I was still very much an adolescent, my character and faith greatly matured over the course of time. I loved being at school—learning new things, seeing the teachers, and being around my friends.

My friends and I frequented each other's houses to hang out and endlessly play video games or get into trouble. My friends and I, like all other guys, had an affinity for fire. We often found something to light on fire or blow up. We didn't destroy our good things, so if we didn't have something to burn, we created something suitable for this purpose. One time Aaron and I built a miniature building framed out of extra plastic flashing from model kits and hot glue; the façade was construction paper. We poured some gasoline on it for good measure. That thing sure burned well, but Aaron and I did not think it through all the way; in the backyard of my suburban home, that sucker put out large billows of dark black smoke!

As I began my sophomore year, my balance continued to worsen. I became increasingly less stable. Eventually walking in the middle of the hallways became too difficult. Navigating from class to class, I walked along the walls, either leaning on them or using them as stabilizers if I started to wobble. Falling down became a more frequent occurrence. Now I knew for sure that my body was acting abnormally. It is a strange thing, at such a point in one's life, to begin to fall down so often. Falling is generally something elderly people worry about, and losing the ability to stabilize myself and prevent falling was hard to reconcile. While I was worried about what may come next, I still relied on God in my frustration and kept living and enjoying life.

One activity which I greatly enjoyed was playing music. With the exception of Matt Klements, all of my good friends and I were members of both the high school symphonic and jazz bands, as well as the pep band. We each played brass instruments. Tyler Olson—my good friend since the eighth grade—and I played trumpet; Aaron the trombone; and Matt Kok, the baritone. Being in these bands, we had concerts and played at football and basketball games.

One night we were at a basketball game, and it was between periods. My friends and I, deciding to take a break, went outside with a few others. I have long since forgotten what the heck we were doing, but some of us started chasing each other in the dark. As I was chasing somebody, I either tripped or lost my balance and fell backward. As I fell, I managed to brace myself by extending one of my arms behind me so that I wouldn't hit my head. I didn't hit my head, but the arm which took the brunt of my weight sure felt weird and I couldn't bend it.

My friends did something of a fireman's carry and took me to the cafeteria where I sat until the game ended. Aaron's mom picked us up from the game that night. She knew I'd broken my arm and didn't look forward to breaking this news to my parents. After returning home, my parents took me to the emergency room, where x-rays showed that not only was my arm broken, but also that I would need surgery the next day to set the bone with pins.

Now, this news didn't worry me at all! I'd had spinal surgery, so arm surgery would be nothing. And it was! The only effort I had to put into all of this had to do with recovery after the cast came off and the pins came out. The anesthesia, however, did make me feel nauseous afterward, but I made sure to hold my vomit until right after I had left the hospital; that way, they wouldn't keep me there any longer!

Because I was down one arm, I decided to have some fun with it. The cast was great because I could smack anything with it and it wouldn't break or hurt my arm. I loved hitting poles, walls, doors, desks, and even friends—though I didn't hit them as hard. I'd broken my right arm, and I am right-handed, so I had to get help for any written assignments. This was very nice! I am not ambidextrous, and I did not learn to be. (However, I played Red Alert 3 on the computer quite frequently, and I *did* learn how to navigate the mouse with my left hand...)

But getting back to my arm surgery... The part that really stunk was that I could not play my trumpet, and I had to miss playing in a concert with music that I had practiced and enjoyed playing. My broken arm occurred at an interesting time in our family. My injury really had nothing to do with Friedreich's Ataxia. It was also interesting because quite shortly before I'd broken my arm, my sister Jeanelle had been in a cast with the exact same break in her left arm. The break was due to hyper-extension and we each had torn a tendon which, in turn, took a piece of the humerus with it. It is such an uncommon break, that the doctor threatened to write about my family in a medical journal if my brother suffered the same break!

After however long it took for my arm to mostly set, the doctor cut my cast in two so that he could look at my arm and the pins that held it together. Everything looked good, the halves of the cast were put back around my arm, and the doctor put medical tape around it to keep it together. I was excited, however, because he told me that with the health of my arm and the halves of the cast being taped together, I could take my cast off and show people my arm, with the pins still in it! And that's exactly what I did. When I returned to school, I gathered my friends and started to remove my cast. They were all somewhat squeamish at seeing my arm, but I thought it was cool.

Showing off my arm with all its hardware wasn't the only thing I did for fun. Aaron and I were still in Boy Scouts, and we'd been involved in scouting since elementary school. We went on many campouts and participated in many scouting functions with our troop. We loved these times because we could cause trouble and not get caught. We did things like chopping down a tree at Boy Scout camp, getting another scout in trouble for our throwing chunks of wood down the river while other scouts were practicing canoeing, throwing rabbit pellets into the shorts of our friend during a morning devotional service, and wedging wood into a port-a-potty door and trapping someone inside. These were only a few of our exploits. We had a terrific time in Boy Scouts and in spite of the mischief we caused, we learned many things.

During my sophomore year, I'd earned enough merit badges and completed enough requirements to earn my Eagle Scout award. This achievement required much dedication and work. This effort and process helped me develop leadership skills, strong character, an understanding of the founding principles of the United States, and other life skills. Both Aaron and my brother Daniel also achieved the rank of Eagle Scout.

So during my sophomore year I broke an arm and achieved my Eagle Scout award among other things, but that's not the only way it ended. As I mentioned before, I'd become accustomed to walking close to the walls, and eventually leaning on them for support. But my body started to yet again change for the worse.

Eventually my balance became so poor that in addition to leaning on the walls as I walked, I also found myself looking for anything I could grasp to steady myself. I started to reach for anything that could prevent my falling, whether it be the railings, borderers of bulletin boards on the wall, gaps in walls, or really anything protruding. I employed this technique between classes and in the classroom. I traveled from one piece of furniture to the next holding on to whatever I could find.

It is really something that nothing ever happened in the art room, with perils like the kiln, hot wax, paints, clay, and the occasional puddle of water spilled on the floor during the course of class. By this time, since my balance had become so bad, falling down was a regular thing. I fell at least two or three times a day. I never *really* hurt myself; I guess I got good at falling; I learned how to prevent bad pain or injury.

Though terribly frustrated at times, I continued to live my life as best as I could. It was difficult to experience, in the span of two years, myself going from being able to walk fairly normally to relying on grabbing anything I could reach to keep myself upright. And more changes were about to come.

Chapter 6

A Small Patch of Fat

Summer was a nice break; I didn't have to worry about schoolwork or navigating the halls and classrooms each day. Summer breaks were a good time to hang out with friends and family, and usually go on a family vacation. That summer, between my sophomore and junior years, my family went on a big vacation to London.

I believe it was in July of that summer that I went to yet another doctor, though I don't remember which doctor I saw. At this point, I still received the odd x-ray in order to monitor my spine and make sure the fusion continued to work. They also monitored the lower, non-fused part of my spine to see if it was curving also. Since my spinal fusion surgery 2 1/2 years prior, the x-rays had never shown problems.

Well, I went in, got the x-rays, and waited until the doctor came in with the results. I thought, *Another day another doctor. He will just give me the same news that I've been getting at all my appointments, that my x-rays are normal and my back is fine.* That's what I thought, but with all the changes I was experiencing, it was foolish of me to expect that.

The doctor told my mother and me that my spinal fusion still looked good. The area where I had surgery was fused and was not shifting, but, the unfused lower part of my spine had begun to curve. Unfortunately, that meant I would be required to undergo another spinal fusion surgery to correct it. The second surgery would fuse me from the lower neck to the end of the spine. This was not great news and meant more hospital time and trips to the doctor.

I don't exactly remember how the timeline worked out, but the doctor gave this spiel about the surgery and its possible complications, and said that he could probably get me scheduled for surgery during the summer so that I would not miss any school the next school year. Thus, my parents scheduled a surgery date during the summer, and I did not have much time to mentally prepare for another procedure like that. Having already gone through a spinal fusion once, and knowing that it would not be as invasive of surgery as the first, I was much less anxious about it this time. But, still, I had some anxiety.

Additionally, one thing that the doctor explained that the surgeon might do bothered me, and it must have flown over my head in everything leading up to my previous fusion surgery. During the surgery, they would be working on my spine—which contains the spinal cord.

The doctor said that if the surgical team felt that they had disturbed the delicate and vital spinal cord, with my parents' permission beforehand, they might temporarily wake me up during surgery and ask me to move something to show that they hadn't damaged the spinal cord. Of all the other "ifs" combined with all the things I did know about the surgery and recovery, it was this little precautionary step which scared me the most. I really did not want to have to wake up during the surgery. As the surgery approached, I talked to my parents and, thankfully, they agreed to deny permission for that.

Because I'd "been here, done this" once before, when the day came, it held much less fanfare in my mind than I had experienced during the lead up to previous surgery. In the time preceding the surgery, I, friends, and family continued to pray—either for healing, or for health and safety in the surgery. At least for me, there was much less wariness in my mind.

After the surgery was over, I woke up without any problems. The initial recovery right after surgery was not much different. It was still very painful, and I had to work my way to getting out of bed and being able to move around. While I was in the hospital, I didn't have quite as many visitors as I'd had before because, being in the summer, not nearly as many people knew about it. Still, I had frequent visits from family members and close friends.

I remember one instance when my friend Aaron came to visit. The memory of this visit still amuses me. Perhaps it was my second day in the hospital recovering, and I had some sort of drain hooked up to my incision to expel any fluids or extra blood. I was talking with Aaron and he was next to the bed as I felt dampness underneath me. We called the nurses, and they discovered that the drain had come undone.

Aaron had a front-row seat as the nurses began to take care of the drain and change the sheets. As they lifted me, they exposed not only my back—which was covered in blood, but also my bare, gown-less butt! After this unexpected show, Aaron seemed to be in a mild state of shock. My dad told him something like, "You're David's friend, and getting to see everything today!"

My experience with this surgery was similar to my first surgery. Per usual, I enjoyed the various nurses and did my best to impart my politeness, humor, and courtesy to them. The "parade," as I called it, of medical students seemed more frequent during this round of surgery.

These groups came to observe or talk with me because I have Friedreich's Ataxia—a rare disorder. It was uncommon for students and doctors to observe somebody in the hospital who had this disorder. At times I felt like a guinea pig with so many people stopping by and looking at me through the glass. I didn't care about the men, but still ... in the mind of a teenage boy, I thought that many of those female students were pretty!

There were other similarities to my previous surgery, such as the tedious exercises in my bed and the lingering pain of my back recovering from just being cut into. But there was another specific similarity which I previously had identified as the worst part: the removal of the catheter. It was as bad as I'd remembered and remains my most hated experience of each surgery!

Being in the hospital after my second surgery was a little different from the first time. Whereas when I was in eighth grade when my body was not changing that much, now my balance had considerably worsened. There were physical therapists and other specialists who visited me in my room. These added numbers to the parade of medical students coming to see me.

Before I could be discharged from the hospital, I had to have made progress toward walking around. One of these specialists suggested that I try using a walker. I wasn't sure about it, but she said that it wasn't a traditional walker; it had wheels, brakes, and a seat. I wasn't exuberant about trying it out, but I did, and it worked out well in the hospital. She suggested that this might be something we look into for helping me walk around safely when I returned to school. My parents were very interested in this and were all for anything that could make my life easier while simultaneously reducing the risk of my falling down.

I, however, had a different view. I did not want to be like an elderly person having to use a walker to go anywhere. Sure, I fell frequently, but I didn't want to have to rely on a piece of hardware to keep me mobile. In the past few years, as my balance had worsened, some doctors in the Muscle Clinic had encouraged me to think about procuring a motorized wheelchair to improve my mobility and keep myself from falling down.

My response to that advice: Heck no! I could walk, and would do so until I couldn't. So...a walker... Well, that was a little better than a wheelchair, but I still didn't want it. My parents and I still had weeks to make that decision though, as I still had to recover from my surgery before school started.

After leaving the hospital, recovery at home seemed to be going very well. I went through the joys of trying to get my bowels to return to their proper functionality, the pain of showers and movement, and the side-effects of the hard-core painkillers. I absolutely hate those drugs. I've been on Vicodin, Valium, and a number of other painkillers. They do effectively take pain away well, but they mess with my emotions. Some days I felt amazing, like I could do anything...until the afternoon. Then I'd go downhill, and the drugs just made me feel horrible—the opposite of earlier in the day. I made sure that, whether I was in more pain or not, I would get off of those medicines as quickly as I could.

About the time I accomplished this, I started to vomit—maybe once or twice a day. We hoped that something was simply turning my stomach, and that it would go away soon. It didn't, and the vomiting became more frequent. I absolutely hate to throw up, and doing it so frequently was nightmarish. The nights soon became long as I got less and less sleep because I was throwing up so often.

One morning it got so bad that as I woke up, I felt terribly lightheaded and sickly. My parents took me to a doctor's office where they found that I was dehydrated. They put an IV in me and I spent a number of hours there having my fluids replenished. Apparently, I had vomited so much that it had led to dehydration, so the doctors advised my parents to monitor me at home. Because of all of my vomiting during the night, neither my parents nor I felt comfortable with my sleeping on the first level while everybody else slept on the third.

The solution was for family members to take shifts sleeping in the living room with me. Usually, it was my siblings. They still remind me how horrible it was being down there hearing me retch and throw up. Many times, it would just be the retching without anything coming out. If I burp or belch today, Jeanelle or Daniel will still say, "You're not going to throw up, are you?"

For a day or two after being dehydrated, my parents made sure that I kept drinking water, but it seemed like the more I drank, the more I vomited. I had another horrible night where I vomited incessantly. The next morning, my parents took me to the emergency room, but the doctors couldn't find anything wrong. I wasn't sick, and as the day went on, I was able to accept the slow melt of ice chips and hold liquid down to keep myself hydrated. The hospital kept me overnight, and the next morning I was discharged as I seemed able to hold liquid down.

I went back home, and over the course of the day drank, and threw up, *again*. This time my parents weren't going to mess around, and I returned to the emergency room. As the emergency room doctors fumbled around to try to diagnose me, my mom remembered something about a possible complication of fusion surgery that was mentioned in the pre-op consultation.

A Small Patch of Fat

My parents got ahold of the spinal surgeon's office to confer, and the surgeon had the doctors give me a gastro-intestinal test.

I was given some strange solution to drink that had radiated particles in it. I went inside a machine that took some sort of a live x-ray of my internal organs These particles would show up on the x-ray. In essence, as the liquid they gave me worked its way through my body, it could be tracked by the machine.

This test actually discovered something. The liquid I'd ingested made it all the way to my stomach, but no further. It was sitting in my stomach and not making its way to the small intestine. There was good news and bad news in this. The good news is they finally found out why I couldn't eat or drink. The bad news was that this was a surgery complication and that there would be more vomiting in store for me.

I was diagnosed with Superior Mesenteric Artery Syndrome, or SMA Syndrome; a complication of spinal fusion surgery. This artery runs over the duodenum—the area where the stomach connects to the small intestine. Normally, the artery does not touch that connection, however, due to a patch of fat separates them. SMA Syndrome is caused when during a surgery, the patient loses weight abruptly and that fat layer disappears around the artery, thus, compressing and cutting off the connection between the stomach and small intestine. Basically, I couldn't eat or drink because if I did, food or liquid didn't have any way to go past my stomach; it would just come back up!

This, nobody expected. This wasn't in my thoughts when I was praying, asking for God to help me through my surgery. Now I still had to deal with recovery from the surgery, but also with this awful complication that involved seemingly endless vomiting. I was re-admitted to the hospital and was soon given a PICC line.

The PICC (one of the c's stands for catheter!) line was a small tube that was inserted and ran through a vein in my left arm, eventually ending right above my heart. Through the PICC line, I could be fed and hydrated essentially with lipids—or fats. This solution to SMA Syndrome involved having the PICC line for about a month and being fed through it so that the fatty layer beneath my artery would build back up and un-cinch the connection between my stomach and small intestine. Vomiting would start to go away, but I wouldn't be able to eat or drink by mouth until the fatty layer re-developed.

After being in the hospital for a few days and vomiting so much that I was sore, I was able to go back home. I learned that once I threw up all the liquid in my body and there was no more, my body would start to get rid of brown and green bile from my liver. While this was somewhat disturbing, it was, nonetheless, interesting.

After being home, and starting to regain my appetite, I learned another thing while I was unable to ingest. It's amazing how many food commercials are on TV.! It seemed like the majority of commercials were about food, and all I could do was lick my chops, waiting for the time that I could have food on my tongue and in my belly again.

I began my junior year that fall with the PICC line. Being weak from not having normal sustenance, I missed a few weeks of school. I also had a pump that had to go wherever I went to steadily pump the lipids into me. The equipment was difficult to move around, and that was another reason it was hard to get to school very often. I did attend some partial days though, so that I wouldn't get too far behind.

One afternoon I went to school to do some work. Even though I had some despised chemistry to do, the day was going to be a good day because a girl I had a crush on had agreed to help me with schoolwork for a while after her class. There were about ten minutes until the end of the day, and I was excited to spend some time with her. Mostly due to my fatigue, I suddenly had to throw up. When I got my head out of the trash can, I felt really tired and weak. The teacher—the only other person with me in the room at the time—decided that we'd better call my mom and that I should go home. I left before school ended, but thankfully I did not throw up with the girl there. Of all the times I had vomited, this was the worst! I went home and never got to spend even one minute with the girl that day!

As I think back to that time, I don't really feel that my life was significantly altered in the experiences of living with a PICC line, but I do believe that God was further developing my patience. It was not easy having the desire and the appetite to eat, but being unable to consume anything.

After about a month or so, I was elated to try eating some real food to test whether the PICC line was working or not. Sure enough, I was able to hold some things down! The line was soon removed, and I was able to slowly resume my normal life. To my delight, I could eat and drink again and build up my appetite. To my dismay, however, I also returned to school using a walker.

Chapter 7

Graduating with a Walker

My walker wasn't like a walker for an elderly person. Those walkers are usually small, silver, and equipped with tennis balls. I had one of those (minus the tennis balls) for at-home use after the second surgery. The walker that I used in school and out in public was much *slick*er. It was green and was equipped with hand brakes, big wheels, a basket, and a seat that I could use if I needed to. I was stubborn and always made a point to sit in regular chairs no matter how uncomfortable they were. I suspect, however, that the seat on my walker was utilized more by family, friends, and even teachers than it was used by me.

The aspect about the walker that I didn't like was that prominently displayed on a piece of cloth near the top of the walker was a patch with the name of the company that made it. I don't necessarily like being a walking advertisement, and I certainly didn't want to advertise an accessibility company wherever I went. My family later took a trip to the Pacific Northwest and while visiting the Boeing Company in Everett, Washington, I bought a 747 patch which my dad promptly sewed over the company name.

As I entered my junior year of high school, I was not only recovering from the second spinal fusion surgery as well as the gastrointestinal complication it caused—which led to me missing about the first month of school— but I was also adapting to using a walker to keep myself steady on my feet. Though I hated the idea of being a youthful high school student, having to rely on a walker for mobility, I must admit, it did help. Adjusting to a walker became another small milestone in my life. Though I didn't enjoy having to use a walker to get around, I did start to see its benefits.

For homecoming dance that year, Denver Christian had reserved the best location, in my mind, for such an event: Wings Over the Rockies air museum in Lowry. With my walker enabling me to walk further distances without becoming so fatigued, Aaron and I were able to walk around the whole museum and view all the aircraft before the dance started—a task that would have proved difficult at that time without the walker. I loved high school dances and always made a point to dance with a girl at each. I greatly enjoyed that, but the second highlight that year was being able to look at all the airplanes!

As my junior year went by, many great and fun things went on in my life, but my body continued to slowly degenerate. During the second semester, my body started to expend more energy on simple tasks. Walking from class to class, a brief distance, tired me. The band room was on the second level, and the only access to it was via a staircase. More and more, that became a larger obstacle for me to overcome.

Near the end of the year, the high school symphonic band went on a trip to Branson, Missouri. The trip was a blast. We performed a number of times and had a variety of additional experiences. These included a steamboat excursion, riding go-carts, attending some of the entertainment there, and other activities.

By the time of this trip, my legs had started to weaken and did not hold me up as well or carry me very far distances. The part of the trip which I didn't enjoy was when we went to an amusement park outside of Branson in the Ozarks. The park was hilly, and my dad—who was there as a chaperone—and Aaron and I, didn't walk around much because my legs just wore out too quickly. Fortunately, Aaron and I weren't very keen on amusement parks anyway.

The final weeks of my junior year ended and even though I'd resorted to using a walker, and even though walking was becoming somewhat of a chore, I was determined to keep using my legs until I no longer could. The thought of using a wheelchair was not anywhere in my mind. In the summer between my junior and senior years, I was also fortunate to be able to go on a high school youth group mission trip to Tijuana, Mexico. Though I had to overcome much homesickness—even before leaving, and even though the group leaders were a bit nervous about having the ability to provide for my needs, the trip turned out to be a huge blessing—walker and all!

At the start of my senior year, my legs were in a very different state than in the year previous. I'd become increasingly dependent on the help of others while I was at school. To climb any steps at the school I relied on the help of Matt Kok, Aaron, or Tyler. They extended a bent elbow so that I could lock arms with them and safely traverse up or down the stairs. From this position, they could also catch me if I started to fall. I drove them nuts sometimes, because when I came to a small set of stairs, I preferred to lean on them for support and walk up or down the stairs rather than using the nearby ramp. Eventually, on large staircases, I simply had to sit and scoot my way down them.

When the second semester of my senior year came, things changed even more. My balance had become so bad, and my legs so weak, that the walker I used to aid my mobility started to become difficult to use. Even with the walker, I could no longer walk even short distances without tiring. Additionally, I'd begun to lose my balance, and falling once again became a frequent event.

My teachers, parents, and I worked it out so that somebody who shared my schedule between classes would walk with me and guide me in the hallways to try to prevent me from falling. When necessary, I sat on the seat of the walker and this person would push me to my next class.

My good friends were mostly around to help, but I also had a few other classmates who walked with me. One such classmate was a girl a year below me, and initially, it was hard and embarrassing to accept that kind of help from a lovely girl. Knowing that I was about her age and couldn't walk, I felt somewhat helpless and embarrassed.

I did not date while I was in high school. I would have absolutely loved to, but I was dealing with many fears and insecurities in my head—especially after I started using the walker. Fears about how the opposite sex would view me started to come into my mind.

I pondered whether high school girls—some of whom seemed immature—would want anything to do with a high school guy who used a walker and could barely walk. I thought, *"There are plenty of guys who have the ability to do many more things than I, and girls would just view me as boring because I have less to offer and there is less I am able to do"*. Those and other thoughts related to my disorder and how it influenced the way girls perceived me crept into my head.

I encountered much frustration with that and wondered if God was going to bless my life with a relationship at that time. I did not doubt or turn from God because of this, but I did struggle with it for a long time. I believe it's partly because of my inaction but also God's will, that this didn't come about in high school, but God did have other things going in my favor at the time.

By the middle of my senior year, my body was further deteriorating. My school was starting a "pageant" contest called "Mr. Crusader". The crusader was Denver Christian's mascot. The competition would include dancing, a talent, and a question-and-answer segment. In an unexpected moment of spontaneity—the opposite of my character most of the time—I signed up. I don't know why; none of my friends were participating. This event turned out to be a positive experience in my senior year.

I learned dance moves and performed them in my walker in front of a crowded gym. For my talent, I recruited my friend Matt Kok. We performed the "Dead Parrot" sketch from *Monty Python's Flying Circus* which was met by much laughter. I advanced to the final question-and-answer section, during which I talked about my Grandpa Car, how I would represent the school if I won, and how my character was similar to a cast-iron pan. Out of about twelve contestants, I won the runner-up position! It was a great time.

As school went on, and I continued to struggle with mobility, my history teacher Mr. Posthumus, brought something to school for me. His wife had had some medical needs and had required the use of an electric scooter for a time. Mr. Posthumus brought the scooter to school so that I could utilize it when traveling between classes.

I did not want to have to use a wheelchair, nor did I want to end up dependent on a scooter, but between classes, I used the one Mr. Posthumus provided, and discovered that it was fun! I was surprised at the speeds I could reach on it. The closest I ever came to getting detention was on this scooter!

It was my style to go fast on this scooter, and once as I approached the intersection of two hallways, I lost control a bit and hit the throttle. As I sped across the hallway, I nearly ran over another student! When I made my way to my destination, Mrs. Bull, a Spanish teacher, ran after and told me, "That's the closest I've ever come to giving you a detention!" After that I still went fast, but did so with greater care!

Our band took another trip during my senior year—to Disney World. I didn't always like the walker, but, again, it did have its benefits. One great thing at Disney World was that I got an accessibility pass which meant that, because I did not have the strength to stand for long periods, when I went to a ride, I could go to the front of the line. Not only me, but my friends also! This was also great because I did not want to ride without my group of friends! We were able to go on many rides because of this, and some operators would even let us ride a few times in a row! That was a terrific perk of using a walker!

As the end of the school year drew near, God placed it on my heart that I should speak during a school chapel service, talking about all of my life changes, and how my relationship with Him was impacted by them. I asked permission and was given the go-ahead. One of my great memories of my senior year was that chapel service.

I felt very fortunate to share my testimony with my school and to boast in my weaknesses, and therefore in the Lord's strength. The Lord is great! Being able to share that amid the context of hardship, which I was still very much dealing with every day, was a tremendous experience.

The school year came to a close, and graduation was quickly approaching. At the school awards ceremony, where I didn't usually receive anything because my academics were not stellar, I was given the Outstanding Senior Boy of the Year award. This award was given to a senior, based on having a mature Christian lifestyle, being involved in multiple activities, academics, and respected by staff and fellow students. I felt shocked and blessed to receive such a recognition. Even so, I recognized that what led to this award and how people viewed me and my life were the result of God's work in me, and not anything I had done. My personality and my character would be very different if I did not have Christ in my life.

Graduation came and it was an exciting time. As I crossed the stage to get my diploma I leaned on my walker. I received a Bible and my diploma. High school, where I'd grown and learned so much, had now ended.

Chapter 8

Endings to New Beginnings

I wrote lengthily on my years in high school because that time greatly shaped my life. Through the course of those four years, I observed and experienced the rapid failing and deteriorating of my body. I went from being able to walk with some wobbles, to leaning on the walls as I walked, to clinging to the walls to keep me upright, to depending upon the support of friends and classmates to navigate between classes, to having to rely on a walker for mobility, to graduating with a walker, awful balance, and weak legs.

For anybody of any age, these would be terrible life circumstances. Though it was hard to lose certain abilities and to be unable to participate in many things most high school students participate in, I came out of that time at peace. Absolutely I got terribly frustrated at times during those years, but I never took it out on God.

These experiences only matured my faith and convinced me that I am loved by my Creator. Though my life may be difficult—not only with my physical trials, the Lord has a plan for me and I had seen that He could use my hardships for His glory in my life and in the lives of those around me.

Through that time, I was also humbled. I, myself—and probably most other people— did not want to have to rely on the help of others in my life. I didn't want help doing what I felt one should have been able to do at that age, and I didn't want to waste other people's time if I did need help. I was brought to a point where I really had no other choice than to accept help from others.

At times, I had so many people wanting to help me, but I simply wouldn't accept their help. It took a number of years, but I learned to graciously and humbly accept help even when I didn't necessarily want it, but recognized that I needed it. Self-advocacy is something that I've gotten better at, but can still struggle with.

With high school over, the time for college was approaching. Having seen my body go downhill over the past four years, I wondered what may come in the next few years. Would I see much more decline? What was in store for my future?

Truths I've Experienced

Strength in Weakness

> Therefore, in order to keep me from becoming conceited, I was given a thorn in my flesh, a messenger of Satan, to torment me. Three times I pleaded with the Lord to take it away from me. But he said to me, "My grace is sufficient for you, for my power is made perfect in weakness." Therefore, I will boast all the more gladly about my weaknesses, so that Christ's power may rest on me. That is why, for Christ's sake, I delight in weaknesses, in insults, in hardships, in persecutions, in difficulties. For when I am weak, then I am strong.
>
> 2 Corinthians 12: 7-10

How is it that I am able to live with a body which has fallen, and continues to fall apart, gives me ire almost each day, and yet take joy in my circumstances and view my physical disorder as a blessing? I have a number of reasons. But specifically, what encouragement do I have in such seemingly dreary circumstances?

Some of my favorite verses in the Bible come from 2 Corinthians, and I love 2 Corinthians 12: 7-10 because it is so relevant to my life. In this chapter, I will dissect this passage, and put it back together in full at the end. In this epistle, Paul is defending his ministry and apostleship. As he goes on, he speaks about revelations that God has shown him. He writes in verse 7, "Therefore, in order to keep me from becoming conceited, I was given a thorn in my flesh, a messenger of Satan, to torment me."

The Lord had given special visions to Paul. To keep Paul humbled and to keep him from thinking highly or haughtily of himself because of what had been revealed to him, he was given a thorn in the flesh. It seems that Paul developed some sort of physical malady. Maybe, maybe not; apparently it's not important for us to recognize exactly what Paul's "thorn" was. This thorn in Paul's flesh would cause him troubles, but also served to keep him from being stuck-up.

Paul continues in verse 8, "Three times I pleaded with the Lord to take it away from me." While this acknowledges and signifies the trouble this malady caused in Paul's life, it also reveals his faith and his confidence that the Lord has the power to heal. Verse 9 further explains Paul's situation:

> "But he said to me, 'My grace is sufficient for you, for my power is made perfect in weakness'. Therefore, I will boast all the more gladly about my weaknesses, so that Christ's power may rest on me."

God reminded Paul that the gift of grace through Christ's death and resurrection, and the love God demonstrated through that was all Paul needed in order to deal with his thorn. Not only that, but the Lord told Paul that His power is made perfect in weakness. Think about all of the things in the history of the world: of nations, of survival, of sicknesses, of injuries, of the animal kingdom, etc. In these areas and others, when has weakness ever been better than strength? I'm hard-pressed to think of a single example. Yet God, the Almighty Creator, whose power knows no bounds has decided to use weakness to display strength. If you really think about it, that seems astronomically contrary to how a powerful God would reveal His glory to and through humanity. This mystery of God has always confounded me, but at the same time, as a Christian, it does make great sense to me.

Where would unbelievers, if they were to believe in God, expect power to be displayed? They would expect, as many expected of the Messiah, that God would plainly show himself and display great power and strength among mankind. They would not expect to find God's strength shown through the weakness of a mortal being.

Think about somebody you know, perhaps yourself, who has had hardship after hardship to deal with. If the particular individual is a believer, perhaps he or she has been able to handle troubles extremely well and display amazing fortitude. That is God's strength shining through weakness—displaying the hope all can have in salvation, promising to us that better times are ahead and that God will work in and through the hardship. You may know somebody who deals with troubles and who may have a good attitude but who does not believe in God. I believe it's possible for people to build up some motivation and strength within ourselves, but I can attest to this: whatever bit of strength I have been able to conjure up lasts for but a short time. With eternal hope, that encouragement is rooted deeply in one's soul.

Paul ends this passage by saying, "That is why, for Christ's sake, I delight in weaknesses, in insults, in hardships, in persecutions, in difficulties. For when I am weak, then I am strong." Paul shares an important point here.

Does this verse ring a bell in your mind:

"When you have faith in Christ, you will lead a continually joyous life, free of trouble and sadness and pain." I hope you do not recognize that because IT'S NOT IN THE BIBLE! Becoming a Christian doesn't mean that life will get easier!

Let's look at the real verse—Jesus' words spoken to his disciples in John 16:33 "In this world, you will have trouble. But take heart! I have overcome the world." Here's a dose of reality: God Himself lets us know that we will all face trials, sin and death are certainties, *and* His grace is sufficient for us.

In 2 Corinthians 12:10, Paul brings up a good point. Weaknesses come in a multitude of forms. The troubles we face can be of our own making, or can be difficulties wrought by the actions of others. They can also be random occurrences—such as a double inheritance of a recessive gene. These verses in 2 Corinthians make it clear that the thorn in the flesh is as applicable to your life as it is to anyone's.

You may never have had a physical malady, but there's been something in your life that has brought, or even now brings, you struggle. Your thorn may be a relational problem between family members or friends. It may be trouble at work. It may be a sickness or disorder, abuse of some form that you've gone through, an addiction you have developed, or some other type of emotional or mental anguish. Thorns can take on many forms, the possibilities are endless.

Paul also says to delight when you are insulted and persecuted because of Christ. As for persecution itself, that is a whole topic on its own. I hardly have any experience with it, but this verse says that along with trials we face, we are to also take joy while experiencing persecution as a Christian.

In my life, my physical disorder isn't the only trial I have faced, even though it is usually the most significant. The reality is that Jesus Himself said that we will all face trouble in life. But, through His death and resurrection, Jesus completely conquered at that moment, for time and all eternity, sin and evil and the grave. And the Lord promises to help us through our times of trial when we face them. God's grace is sufficient for us; when we have such hope for our next life and have received His grace, what really is there to worry about when we face hardship?

The last part I want to briefly expand upon from these verses is in the Lord's response, "for my power is made perfect in weakness." I mentioned the seemingly opposing notions of power in weakness. When considered further, sense can be made of this. I've often heard the adage which states, "God won't allow us to go through more than we can handle." I have heard this, and used to believe that, it, but as I grew older and read the Bible in more detail and context, I learned that it makes sense that God *would and does* allow us to go through times in our lives during which we do not have adequate strength. I also discovered that this adage is *not* a verse in the Bible. It is often confused and is sometimes equated with 1 Corinthians 10:13. This verse states:

> "No temptation has overtaken you except what is common to mankind. And God is faithful; he will not let you be tempted beyond what you can bear. But when you are tempted, he will also provide a way out so that you can endure it.

However, upon reading the actual verse and writing before it, it is clear that Paul is talking about temptations, not about trials. And the two are very different things.

When I learned this, I was somewhat disheartened. But after my initial thoughts, I took hope in finding that the verse did not promise that God would "protect" me from my times of trial. (Because I have had trials that are seemingly too difficult for me to handle!) I've learned in my life, not only with my physical trials, but also in dealing with other trials and temptations, that my strength is very little to none.

Again, I believe it's possible for all of us to muster some strength or motivation in our lives, but if we rely solely on that, it fizzles rapidly. I've often been told what a great attitude I have and what a great outlook on life I display, but that credit is not due to me. It's because of the way I've been molded, and, actually thanks in large part to the very troubles I have gone through. Of course, God wants to allow us to face trials that we cannot handle on our own! If we could handle them ourselves, why would we ever need His help?

The Lord wants us to rely on Him when life seems hopeless. People need God because our strength is so small. God's power is made perfect in weakness; He can use the worst times to bring us the most blessing and His glory can be revealed in you even during your worst circumstances. God is faithful and will help us during our times of hardship. His glory can be revealed to the world and witnessed by unbelievers through the attitudes, worldviews, joy, and happiness of Christians whose lives seem to be more difficult or of less quality than the average person. His power is made perfect in weakness through our reliance on Him in those times.

Growing older and experiencing the changes my body has gone through since the time of the diagnosis to the present—in which my body, and indeed, my life itself, continues to be dynamic—I take joy in knowing that I do not have to be in control of taking care of my needs, of managing every new challenge. I can trust in God to watch over me. He is my comfort. He gives me strength. In many ways I am weak, and my body is certainly weak—though not of my choosing. Yet in my faults, and in my weaknesses, I am completely enabled! I am weak, but through my faith and God's grace, I am strong.

> Therefore, in order to keep me from becoming conceited, I was given a thorn in my flesh, a messenger of Satan, to torment me. Three times I pleaded with the Lord to take it away from me. But he said to me, "My grace is sufficient for you, for my power is made perfect in weakness." Therefore, I will boast all the more gladly about my weaknesses, so that Christ's power may rest on me. That is why, for Christ's sake, I delight in weaknesses, in insults, in hardships, in persecutions, in difficulties. For when I am weak, then I am strong.
>
> 2 Corinthians 12: 7-10

Chapter 9

An Endearing Rule

The time after high school began with melancholy. I was glad to be finished with high school, but for 13 years I'd been going to school with the same friends and classmates and had developed great relationships with my teachers as well. Now all that was going to change, but such is life.

I enjoyed my final summer with my friends before we all went our separate ways. The hardest goodbye was to Aaron, my best friend since kindergarten. He'd been accepted to the United States Merchant Marine Academy in King's Point, New York. We had done so much together, and now we would be able to see each other only infrequently.

I again, for the second and final time, was able to go on the high school youth group trip to Mexico. Aaron could not go on this trip, but my other friends did and we had much fun and enjoyed interacting with the kids at Vacation Bible School. It was another fulfilling week of service to God, and it was hard to leave.

What made it even harder to leave was that two lovely Mexican girls my age had gotten to know me some, gotten my contact information, and were sad to see me leave—one even cried! With the "girls" situation in my life, I thought, *dang, maybe I should move to Mexico, I may have better chances here!*

I returned from the mission trip in July. I ended my summer by saying further goodbyes and looking ahead to what college may bring. I'd been accepted to Colorado Christian University (CCU). Thankfully they accepted me, as that was the only school to which I had applied!

Colorado Christian University is in Lakewood, Colorado, and the campus is not especially large. This would also be beneficial because with my difficulty getting around, I wouldn't have to travel long distances to get from place to place. This was important because near the end of high school and through the following summer, walking had become much more difficult for me.

I continued to be stubborn, walking even though my energy drained very quickly. I went to the Muscle Clinic for the last few times. I'd turned 18 and had aged out of the clinic at the Children's Hospital will. During my last visits they encouraged me to try out an electric wheelchair. My parents began to think this may be a good idea for my time in college, so we went to a store where these chairs were sold. I sat in one and tested it out, and like the scooter, I found it to be very fun, but not for full-time use.

After arriving home, my parents and I discussed the wheelchair. We considered the need to regularly charge it at school. We also discussed the weight of the thing ... its advantages and disadvantages.

Each time I thought about having to rely on an electric wheelchair, I seriously felt a sick feeling in my stomach. I suppose much of that was pride and probably some form of grief, but I genuinely did not see the need to give up walking and instead get around by pushing the joystick of an electric wheelchair with my fingers even though I was still able and had a strong upper body. I feared losing my strength if I wasn't using those muscles.

After much back and forth, I eventually brought up an idea that had been in the back of my parents' minds: I told them that I would be much more comfortable trying out a manual wheelchair. That way I could use my arms and still exercise while I moved, and it would also solve some of the logistical problems of having a motorized wheelchair at college. I had also planned to continue to live at home and commute to school, so a huge bulky chair didn't make sense in the lower level of the house anyways. I also conceded that if the manual chair did not work out, I would try the electric model. Another big change in my life had come, and I started college as a reluctant user of a wheelchair.

Thankfully, the campus was fairly easy to traverse. Many of the buildings were close to each other. There were some hills, so I could get exercise on the way up and have fun on the way down!

Though I didn't like this new experience of meeting people from the vantage point of a wheelchair, getting around was easier and saved more energy than walking with the walker. Not living on campus, not liking change, and not having had to make new friends for 13 years, I found it difficult for quite a while to get to know people in college.

Also, having to adjust to life in a wheelchair, had me feeling somewhat insecure. I came to learn that there are, of course, many good and nice people who are not at all uncomfortable around a person who uses a wheelchair. However, there are also many who don't know how to deal with someone who uses a wheelchair, and that either the wheelchair or their lack of experience around people with disabilities pushes many away.

Additionally, I felt the sting of dismissal (and frequently of not even having been acknowledged) each time others spoke only with the person pushing the wheelchair and focused solely on that person while completely ignoring the occupant of the chair.

However, through many years in college, I learned a very valuable lesson. Sometimes, the wheelchair attracted people's attention, particularly the ladies'. One year, the location of a course in which I was enrolled required me to climb a large hill to get to the class. I could certainly get up the hill, it just took some time. The weight distribution made it so that my chair constantly popped up on two wheels as I turned the wheels to carry myself forward uphill.

As I did this one day, a pair of girls, whom I could not see as they were behind me, didn't merely offer to push, but instead told me they were going to help me up the hill and also that they would do this on each day that we shared a similar schedule. When we got to the building and on flat ground one of them held open the door, and I saw these two gorgeous girls!

I was in utter shock and jubilation as these girls told me they would regularly be helping me! I was filled with glee, that they would do this each time I ran into them! Certainly, after this, I had made myself a golden rule: if a lovely lady ever asks me if I'd like help and offers to push me how, I should always say yes!

To my consternation, I broke my own rule a few times, but that was the exception. This rule worked tremendously while in college, as there were numerous ladies around who offered to help me. However, my rule did have one downside, and here it is: I could not see the person who was pushing me! I suppose I could have turned my head or lifted it straight up to look behind me, but that would've looked awfully strange. Even so,

I loved being pushed in my chair by young ladies, and I enjoyed their company.

As I get older, hopefully ladies will still see me and offer to help me, and not see me as creepy! I have found this an endearing rule to live by, and although spontaneous offers of assistance do not come with as much frequency anymore, the rule still applies and has paid off since college.

Truths I've Experienced

Worry

So do not worry, saying, 'What shall we eat?' or 'What shall we drink?' or 'What shall we wear?' For the pagans run after all these things, and your heavenly Father knows that you need them. But seek first His kingdom and His righteousness, and all these things will be given to you as well. Therefore do not worry about tomorrow, for tomorrow will worry about itself. Each day has enough troubles of its own."

Matthew 6: 31-34

The reason my views in life are contrary to my circumstances is because God's Word promises help in times of trouble in this life, and tremendous blessings in the next. I've explained how God promises help through difficult periods in life to those who love him. Part of putting trust in God is not fretting about what may come.

In the above passage, excerpted from the Sermon on the Mount, Jesus instructs His disciples not to worry about the future, and reminds them that nothing good comes of such concern. This is a terribly difficult concept for everybody on the planet to grasp. Worrying is something everybody does; it is a part of human nature and it is easy to do.

When you turn your life to Christ however, you are given the command and the ability to cease dwelling on the unknown. Like everybody else, I have plenty that I can worry about. Bad moods and fatigue can incessantly increase my mind's wandering. Unlike most people, my body is not in a normal state, and falling into speculation of what may come of my body in the years to come can be quite easy.

Allow me to give some disclosure of the forms of certain worries I have had. Since diagnosis, I have had worries about my body in the future. How much more will my body change? To what lengths will it deteriorate? Will more changes happen within the next three years, months, or many years from now? Could I go blind eventually? Will it lead to, or hasten, my death? Could I lose the ability to use my hands? Will I end up being unable to do anything for myself? Will I have further heart problems? Will I have a stroke? Will I end up in a motorized wheelchair? With my limitations, will it be difficult to find a girl attracted to me? Will I be able to get married? Will I have the joy of being a father, and if so, how much would I be able to do with my kids? Whether it's me on my own or with family support, will I be able to acquire a job that will provide for my needs and for the needs of my family should that be a part of my future?

These and numerous other worries plague my thoughts. Like anybody else, my worries focus on the future, and the many unknowns that lie ahead. What is God's plan for me in this lifetime? I don't know, but I love reading this part of the Sermon on the Mount and gleaning encouragement from it because the act of worrying is detrimental. God doesn't want us putting our energy into worries because doing so can hold us back. It may keep us from action, from effort, from speaking up, from serving, and from doing God's will. Worrying plays to our fears and only does harm.

Satan wants us to worry and seeks to burden us with it. No good comes of worrying. Worry is an effective tool to cripple people. This is why God wants us to quit worrying! And Jesus talks about worrying—or rather about NOT worrying—in Matthew. He makes it sound very easy to simply not worry.

At times in our lives, it can be simple to trust God's provision. But most times, our fallen nature makes that very difficult. There have been times in my life where my faith compelled me to completely put my trust in the Lord for my future. Other times it is difficult to conquer my mind and emotions and put my full faith in God.

Christian life is a flux, and while I am certainly not perfectly successful in abolishing worry from my life, each day I do believe that God plays an active role in my life and that He will take care of me in my future. As a Christian, I'm not promised comfort or pleasure in life, but I know above the foolishness of my mind, that He looks out for my best interests.

I've also found another effective tool against worry. It is from a passage in the Bible I haven't heard preached about much, but it gives an important lesson. At the beginning of 1 Samuel, the Israelites, as is typical for all of us, again rebelled against God. God turned His face and allowed the Philistines to defeat them. The Israelites pleaded with the prophet Samuel, repented, and turned back to the Lord. Samuel, having prayed, told the people to gather at a place called Mizpah, where he would intercede for them. When the Israelites went to Mizpah, the Philistines attacked. With Israel repentant towards Him, God thundered and threw the Philistines into a great panic, causing them to flee and lose the battle.

The Israelites, suddenly victorious, chased and routed their attackers. Then Samuel took a stone and set it up between Mizpah and Shen. He named it Ebenezer, saying, "Thus far the Lord has helped us." 1 Samuel 7:12. The meaning of the name Ebenezer is "stone of help." Samuel established this marker not only in praise to the Lord for helping Israel in that battle, but for remembrance. When Israelites would later pass by Ebenezer, they would see it and remember, *that stone signifies the Lord's deliverance of Israel from the Philistines at Mizpah, He is faithful.*

The concept of the Ebenezer stone has played an important part in my life. It can be easy to fall into worry and anxiety, but a great way to combat this is to remember God's faithfulness. If I slow down and dwell on the help, the comfort, the blessings the Lord has given me in my past, it becomes harder to worry. When focusing on God's love and faithfulness—how He's always been with me to help me, that He promises never to leave me—then my love for Him and my trust in Him grow exponentially.

This concept holds true not only in reminding me of God's faithfulness in past trials, but also simply in all of my daily thoughts. In Philippians 4:8, Paul says,

> "Finally, brothers and sisters, whatever is true, whatever is noble, whatever is right, whatever is pure, whatever is lovely, whatever is admirable—if anything is excellent or praiseworthy—think about such things."

Like the Ebenezer stone reminds us of God's faithfulness, I can certainly confirm that if my thoughts are on the good things like in the above passage, my outlook changes for the positive. This is compared to thinking about worries, which only brings negativity.

There is, however, an unfortunate reality associated with this. Because I'm a sinful being, I easily get distracted and occupied, and many times when my mind wanders into wrong places, I do not take the time to ponder and remind myself of God's faithfulness in my past. I yearn that I would do the opposite more often! There is no shortage of examples of God's faithfulness in my life!

Worry is a false force that is used against us to prevent us from accomplishing greater things, but when you take the time to dissect your past and focus on God's faithfulness in your personal life, then you will notice your anxiety being swept away. Sadly, since we are humans, worrying will never be completely eradicated in this lifetime, but we have been given tools and promises from God to keep them at bay when we face them.

Chapter 10

CCU, DC, & NY

During my third year at Colorado Christian University, I was afflicted with intense anxiety, and it wasn't even due to my own body. My sister Jeanelle had graduated and left for college in Seattle. For some reason, I became completely overwhelmed with anxiety and worry at that time. My thoughts affected my eating, sleeping, and free time. Still living at home, I worried about the changes that would take place there. Since I could remember, Jeanelle, Daniel, my parents, and I had all lived in the same household. Now Nell was gone. For some reason, her absence sparked irrational fears and what-if scenarios in my mind.

Eventually, these anxieties grew to concerns about other people in my family. The devil chose this time in my life to pollute my mind with ridiculous worries and I can't say exactly why, other than for the purpose of adding further angst into my life at that time. Through this time, I prayed, and prayed, and prayed.

I'd never faced anything like this before in my life. As mentioned previously, it was a strange period in my life that lasted a few months, and I'm not sure how or why it ended, but it showed me that I can't let worries and anxieties hijack my mind and affect my life. This is another reason that I don't focus on my maladies and what may come up concerning them in the future. Taking to heart Jesus' instruction in Matthew 5, I aim not to worry about tomorrow because today has enough troubles of its own.

As I went through college, I slowly discovered that using the wheelchair wasn't all bad. If I went to a baseball game or other events, I would get a good seat with an unobstructed view. Also, most people are courteous and will clear space for a person passing by in a wheelchair.

Some don't, and that is to their own peril! I developed another system that still applies today. If I am trying to get past someone and say, "Excuse me," and have tried to get their attention, yet they remain oblivious, I run into them, gently. This works great because 99% of the time the person looks back with irritation to see what has hit them and when they see it is someone who uses a wheelchair, they feel badly, apologize, and step aside. It is a wonderful system.

A wheelchair can be a good thing at events where I want to meet people, as well. I used to go to many Western Conservative Summits, which CCU's think tank, the Centennial Institute, put on each summer. It is a collection of leaders, politicians, and thinkers speaking about the state of the country. At these events I liked to meet the speakers whom I admire. The wheelchair afforded me a distinct advantage here. I'm in a large, but smaller demographic of people, because most people can walk. When I go up to try to meet somebody, the wheelchair draws their eyes and eventually they gravitate towards me, sometimes going out of their way to meet me. In this way the wheelchair attracts people towards me.

No matter what you think of her, a number of years ago being in a wheelchair helped give me the opportunity to speak briefly with Sarah Palin. She was in a hurry to leave the venue, but she made a point to come over to me, give me a hug, chat for a minute, and introduce me to her husband! Being in a wheelchair can make a person stand out, and not always in a bad way!

In school I oscillated between dabbling in History, then in Youth Ministry, and eventually landed upon Global Studies. Global Studies covered many areas: history, religion, politics, economics, among other topics of study. CCU didn't have a political science major while I was there, otherwise that is what I would have studied, but Global Studies was the closest thing. Being at another small school was great because I saw familiar faces fairly often, and I could develop relationships with professors and other faculty.

One of my favorite places at CCU was an office called the Life Directions Center (LDC). The LDC is where the student advisors were. I went there often to take my tests and exams. This allowed me to develop good relationships with many people there including my own advisor, Jason Makowsky.

Eventually I got a job in the LDC; I kept track of each student's ministry/service hours, of which 180 were required for graduation. I had so much fun there, and it was my favorite place on campus. Jason and I eventually began taking lunches during the week where we would put movies in at the conference table and watch them on the big projector screen. Many days we watched Mr. Bean—my absolute favorite comedic character!

Toward the end of college, I was given the opportunity to go on a few trips. These later proved to be a huge blessing to me. My school had decided to take a group of about 12 students on a trip to Washington D.C. to meet with different people and to speak about relevant topics. I decided I would like to go, so I signed up.

My parents were a bit nervous, as I'd never gone on a trip the length of a week unaccompanied by someone whom I knew well to help me. I certainly was not sheltered, and I was at that time already an adult, so trusting that it would all work out somehow, I decided to go.

It was a tremendous trip. Our group got to tour the Capitol with a senator and enjoyed a meal in its Senate Dining Room. Among other things, we also visited the Dutch Embassy and went to the Pentagon—even attending a devotional service there. Additionally, we went on a tour of DC one night in the rain. A fellow student in my group decided to piggy-back me around the Marine Corps Memorial rather than assisting me in my chair. I excitedly agreed, and the reason for this arrangement was that sitting in my chair in the rain would only have made me wetter from the puddle that would accumulate in my seat. I still got wet—though only on my back.

One of my favorite experiences to look back on happened during that trip. After arriving in DC, a number of students decided to find some food. We were famished because we had not eaten all day. After eating, some people in our group decided to go to the dorm and relax while myself and others decided to explore while the sun was still up. Somehow, probably by choice, I ended up in a group of about five girls. I was the only guy. How horrible was that?

We decided to head towards the American History Museum. As we walked from the museum at which we'd eaten, we came to a small set of three or four stairs. The ramp to by-pass the stairs was a distance away. Not really knowing any of these girls very well, I somehow convinced one of them to take me down the stairs in the chair. I have a terrific photo of my friends from that moment: Chrysandra stood at the top watching with an expression of mixed terror and nervousness, while Sarah, with mixed nervousness and laughter, guided me down the staircase. A passerby in the background had a look of confusion and disgust on her face!

That wasn't the only adventure that day. In the American History Museum, we saw (among other things) the Star-Spangled Banner. Next, we went to the Washington Monument. Chrysandra then wanted to see the White House, and as we headed that way, we encountered another accessibility challenge. Well, the accessibility, itself, was not the challenge. The challenge was of our own creation. Rather than travel the distance to the ramp which led to the lower sidewalk, I suggested we take a shortcut. Yet again I somehow convinced these girls of the benefits of my idea. I slid off my chair, had them lower it to the sidewalk while I sat on the wall—which was about three feet tall. Then, with their help, I lowered myself into the chair from the height of the wall. No problem. From there, we went to the front of the White House and up to the fence. From this vantage, we admired the structure and took pictures of it. Charity pointed out the statue of Andrew Jackson, which she wanted to see, in the park across Pennsylvania Avenue.

"Oh, yeah! Let's go do that!" I exclaimed. I began to briskly push the wheels on my chair, not realizing that the sidewalk was curbed and ending. I took a dive and ended up on the street with my chair toppled over near me. Thankfully, that part of Pennsylvania Avenue was not open to vehicles!

After I fell, all the girls were quite concerned, arousing the attention of several police who rushed to my aid. They helped me back into my chair and were quite worried about any possible injuries.

My only injury was a scrape on my elbow. Not even my pride was wounded. I thought, *Of all places to fall out of my chair, in front of the White House is a decent place!* Later, I was disappointed that I neglected to have somebody take a picture of me crashed on the street in front of the White House; I would've admired that picture! After I was situated in my wheelchair, the police gave me some iodine—which I didn't think I needed—to put on my road rash—but, oh well. We decided to start heading to the dorm because it was beginning to get dark. The girls were still amped up because of what happened, but it was no big deal.

This day of adventure was almost over and Chrysandra pushed me in my wheelchair as we were going back. We hit a crack in the sidewalk which the little front wheels of my chair could not handle and I went flying out of the chair once more. The girls were able to help me get up, but, thinking it her fault, Chrysandra was afraid to try to help me anymore. I found it hilarious. At that time, falling was fairly commonplace when family or friends pushed me in my wheelchair or walker. Usually, mishap was caused more by me than by the operator!

After this, we returned to the dorm without further incident. It had been quite a day: While making new friends, I had (safely) descended a staircase in my chair, practically rappelled down a wall (again safely), dumped myself in front of the White House (acquiring only a scrape), and been ejected once more (also safely). I look back at that and think, *What a great day!* Yes, I had fallen and roughed myself up a bit, but that was no big deal. The big deal to me was that I made friends in true David-fashion, and my new friends attested to seeing the glory of God reflected in my attitude that day.

Less than a month after that trip, I was accepted to travel to Long Island, New York to attend an economic seminar. This trip was a bit different then the DC trip, as from my school only I and three other guys attended. Though I further learned on this trip to be more independent, I still had to rely on others to help me out. I had fun on the trip and on the few visits to Manhattan. I even got to see my friend Aaron while I was there.

I had turned 21 that previous May, a month before this trip, so Aaron and I decided to meet at a bar. I had never drunk any alcohol before this, so I had a beer. I was surprised at the number of bathroom trips I had to make! On top of that, not having had alcohol before, I had a buzz, and the different motor signals in my body were all messed up. I was fine but soon learned that having a drink is not something to overdo!

I returned to the hotel and slept off the alcohol. I didn't have a hangover the next day and am glad I was spared that experience. I attended the remaining lectures over the next few days before returning to Colorado. This trip gave me increased confidence in my ability to do more for myself by myself.

Chapter 11

Unwelcomed News

At the end of the summer, my final year of college began, I woke up one morning and started my daily routine to get ready to go to class. That particular morning, however, I felt very sickly in such a way I had never felt before. I didn't have much energy and felt just awful. My parents looked at me and saw that I did not look right.

Starting to worry, my dad took me to the emergency room where they worked to diagnose what was wrong. It did not take long for the medical team to discover that my heart rate was in the upper 100s! For an unknown reason, my heart had gone into an irregular rhythm which I found out could lead to stroke or, at its worst, death. To everyone's relief, I had gone to the hospital right away, thereby decreasing the potential for the risks I mentioned, among others. I was given some sort of medication to regulate my heart rate. My heart slowed to normal, and I felt much better.

The puzzling thing was that for the past few years I had occasionally been examined by a cardiologist, having my heart routinely checked, to make sure that none of the aforementioned possible heart symptoms of Friedreich's were appearing. In those appointments, there had been no indications of any problems. My heart had always seemed fine. I simply have an irregular heartbeat. But what I was experiencing at that time, was something new altogether.

The rapid heart rate that I experienced that particular morning was the first sign of a problem. I ended up in the hospital overnight and most of the next day. When I left, I had a new regimen of heart medication—the same medicine that I had been given in the emergency room to regulate my heartbeat.

This episode was one of the scarier experiences in my life. I had dealt with various forms of degeneration, but I always felt that I still maintained some amount of control over the muscles in my body. My legs grew weaker, but I could still use them, and I could still exercise my other weaker body parts to try to keep the muscles strong. But this was different. The heart is such a vital part of the body, so vital to life. When my heart, an involuntary muscle, decided to speed up, it was not something I could simply tell to slow down!

Through this experience, my reliance was on God. Where else could it be? Certainly not on the medication! No doubt the medicine was working, but medicine bears no guarantee. After this, I saw the cardiologist who found that I had developed Atrial Fibrillation, commonly referred to as AFib. AFib is a heart condition in which the heart can go out of regular rhythm—possibly leading to blood clots and strokes.

This was a symptom of Friedreich's I was hoping not to develop. I didn't want my heart to be affected by my disorder. Not only did I receive this unwelcomed news, but I also learned that if the AFib worsened, I might need a surgery in which a defibrillator would be placed on my heart. This device would shock and attempt to reset my heart whenever it would go into an irregular rhythm.

Thankfully at that time, the medicine worked and nothing further was necessary. As if I did not have to rely on God about my body before... This certainly added to that dependence. I have had all kinds of other things going on with my body, but now heart issues were added to the list.

Even though more frustration and fear abounded, I was not completely dismayed. I'd already been living with a daily physical trial. In the grand scheme of things, what was one more thing to add to the struggle? Learning this terrible news ultimately led to me putting more trust in God. It could be said that I'm stubborn, because as bad as things have gotten, I've chosen to stick with God, not abandon Him. It is a choice I have not regretted.

Truths I've Experienced

On my Disability

> He gives strength to the weary and increases the power of the weak.
>
> Isaiah 40:29

Christians are called to serve their neighbors. And they are especially called to help the less-fortunate. As I look forward and consider my future, I am unsure where, specifically, God wants me. I would love to serve in any ministry capacity, potentially affiliated in some way with the disabled community. Though if that were to happen, it would be an adjustment for me, because I haven't really considered myself a member of that community. I have never wanted to be associated with the term "handicapped" or "disabled," even now that those descriptions are becoming more apparent as time moves forward.

I'm sure the reason for thinking of myself as not involved in that community is probably pride along with the notion that I have never defined myself by my physicality. If I want to do something, I figure out a way to do it. My friends and family have never treated me differently or kept me from pursuing my interests because of my body. However, I'm not one of those people who would take offense if someone referred to me as handicapped or disabled. That would be political correctness, and I absolutely hate political correctness! I am a grown man, and don't care if some use words that I myself don't usually choose to use to describe my reality.

Many people with disabilities are sensitive about the language used in relation to their situation. I remember one instance in which I went to church with my friend Matt Klements and his family. After we had parked, his dad proceeded to pull my walker out the trunk. As he did, an elderly couple walked by. I heard the gentleman remark to Matt's dad, "I see you have a cripple with you this morning."

At first, I was a bit surprised because that word isn't used very much anymore, but then I started to laugh in my head! I found it funny! I'm sure the man meant nothing derogatory, and that was just another word for accurately describing my reality.

I don't take offense to how people refer to me, unless the reference is meant to offend. Perhaps it is a bit odd, but I feel somewhat discouraged when I've met people and they don't ask about my circumstances, even though I know that they are thinking about them! It's unfortunate that people who don't know me seem to tiptoe around me even though I am happy to talk about my condition and experiences and would delight to share my story and testimony. It's usually a good ice-breaker if people are brave enough to ask.

On the other hand, neither do I want the conversation to center on my circumstances. It drives me nuts when those who have a disability center their thoughts, their conversations, and their focus around it. This is not, of course a vast characterization of everyone in this category. A great many people with different handicaps do not want the focus of everything to be on their struggles. But I have run into some who seem to want to shine the spotlight on their disability. I admit that, at some point in many conversations, my disorder does inevitably come up. I will talk about it if people ask, and it does affect most of my daily decisions, but it is not my focus.

Sometimes, I find myself uncomfortable when I am around those with disabilities. It may sound harsh, but *some* with disabilities have an aire of being in some sort of victimhood class. There is a sense of being "owed" by society because of the way they are and how people have treated them. As I have already noted, few people know how to interact with those who have disabilities. Because of this, in some instances such people make sarcastic comments about how others treat them. Years ago, while travelling on a train with a family member, I met a person who was about my age. This person had some sort of paralysis and had movement only of the head and a few fingers. Though a pleasant enough individual, I felt uncomfortable because I noticed a quickness to take offense.

An older conductor walked by, patted me on the back, and I turned and smiled in acknowledgment. Shortly after the conductor departed, the afore-mentioned fellow traveler remarked to me, "I see that you get the old-people-pats, too." The other traveler indicated annoyance at such treatment. The interpretation this person assigned to the pats was, "I feel bad for you, but I'm glad to see you out and about."

I had never really thought about it, but I've received numerous pats on the back when I'm out in different places. I enjoy acknowledgment, and if the small chit-chat started by a pat is well-intentioned, then so be it! That's a good way to meet people or spark up a conversation! I do not feel badly for myself, and I guess if others do, that's their prerogative, but I'm not going to fall into what I see as this "handicapped thought" of feeling upset because other people may feel badly for me. In my view, that's their problem, not mine.

I have run into various people with disabilities who want to speak only about their physical woes, and how have they've had to adjust their lives to their bodies. Many who have a disability have allowed their identity to be dictated by it. Some people with a disability view their life and circumstances with bitterness. (Unfortunately, this view is not held only by those who have disabilities. Lots of people whose lives seem "perfect" also have a bitter attitude.)

I have encountered a person who, in addition to having a physical disability, has the greater disability of a bitter attitude. I'll tell you about this person.

This person and I have similar physical disabilities, but that's where what we have in common ends. This person freely shares personal thoughts, and opinions about life—particularly about personal difficulties. Being utterly bitter about life and about the manifestations of a particular condition, day-to-day living is an experience this person hates. I understand this to a point, but this person is completely miserable!

Rather than striving for a positive outlook, this person seems to strive for negativity by focusing on their disabilities and inabilities. The ensuing bitterness has led to an evangelistically anti-God stance, and rants about how if there were a God, He's not loving or good or understanding of suffering.

After having considered this perspective, I came away feeling dread and hopelessness. I had to remind myself that dread and hopelessness are feelings which do not relate to my life. The difference between this person and me is simple: Having acknowledged Jesus Christ as Savior, I have both a purpose in life, and a hope in eternity.

The person I described above has rejected our greatest ally—God! Without God one has nothing to live for, and zero hope. The perspective this individual has honed says, "Poor me. I ended up with a bum deal in life!" As my disorder has progressed, I have often thought *What would I be like if God wasn't a part of my life, and how then would I have handled my body failing?*

I have a common recurring answer: I believe I have great potential to be a tremendously miserable person. (Actually, each person alive has this potential.) Without the eternal hope of perfection, what is the point of having a positive attitude? What is the point of persevering? It may sound strange, or crazy to those who struggle with bitterness (and maybe even to many who don't struggle with bitterness), but I look at my disorder as a blessing. At the same time, I also believe that as illnesses and disorders are a result of the fall of mankind and of sin coming into the world, God did not *give* me this disorder, but allowed it into my life.

In life, people with physical maladies or disorders don't have to identify themselves or otherwise center their identities around these difficulties. This is especially true for those who believe. While the disorder or disability remains prominent in the life of the person who has a challenge of this type, much good can be done in the lives of others through it. I believe, and have seen, that other people can see God through such circumstances. This is true not only of physical problems, but also of other kinds of trials. God can use adversities that we handle well to impact others in ways that we might not even know. While this is true, it can be very easy to become selfish in our trials and focus on how bad one's *own* situation is. If you ever fall into this, stop, and truly think about this next point: Somebody always has it worse.

This fact not only reminds me to be thankful, but also keeps me humble in my circumstances. Someone may look at me and notice the following: I can't walk, my coordination is awful, I have heart issues, I can't use my fingers terribly well anymore,' I use a wheelchair, I simply don't have the health and agility that most people have. That person may think that I have a pretty hard life.

My situation certainly isn't easy, and at times I do feel very frustrated. For example, I hate when I'm home alone and somehow, I fall on the floor, and am unable to get back up. I absolutely hate it. And, further, I hate that I have to rely on somebody else to help me do something as simple as getting back into a chair.

Friedreich's is progressive; it will continually get worse. Some days, I do absolutely hate having this disorder! While this is the case, I have much for which to be thankful. I'm thankful that even though I have this disorder, I'm fortunate because I know that my situation could be worse; there are many people that I have both seen and known who live with much worse circumstances than I.

Toward the end of college, I started to take the Access-a-Ride bus to school, and later to work. Access-a-Ride is Denver's metro-area accessible public bus service for individuals who find it difficult to use, or who simply cannot use, the regular bus system. Unlike standard public busses, Access-a-Ride picks people up from their homes and takes them directly to their destinations. Access-a-Ride brought me angst in a number of ways ... but I won't go there!

In these small busses, many of the passengers like to converse. Between the passengers and some of the drivers, trips are usually interesting. But using this service also broke my heart.

I saw people with disabilities from missing limbs to various forms and degrees of developmental delays. From my seat in my wheelchair, I saw these children of God and yearned for their healing.

The vast majority of people I saw on the bus had disabilities or disorders that seemed much more difficult than mine. I have come to thank God for my struggles and for not allowing me to deal with the struggles that others have. I am especially thankful that I don't have the challenges presented by cognitive disabilities or mental disorders.

The knowledge that my situation could be much, much more difficult keeps me grateful. While I am not conceited by how I have learned to view my disorder, I am grateful for how I have felt that God has taught me to see it. Of course, while I'm dealing with this trial and doing my best to use it to try to witness and encourage, there is always an element of sin and pride that ebbs and flows—as may be true for all. I ask God to quell this current!

I desperately try not to compare how I deal with my difficulties to how others deal with their difficulties. I do work hard to maintain a positive view in the midst of my struggles. And I do my best to deal with whatever comes in a cheerful way. I never feel that I am *better* than another because of circumstances that are out of human control.

While the devil is constantly seeking to trip me up in this regard, these low-lying prideful thoughts are always squashed when I think of, or see, someone in less-fortunate circumstances than myself. I don't always have to think of somebody with a physical disorder either. I know a number of able-bodied people in my life, even in family, who have fallen into much worse situations than I hope never to ever deal with.

Life is hard, at times tremendously so. For those who feel stuck in a hole, my advice is to take a good, long look at the people you come across and think hard. I guarantee you that someone you know or meet has it a lot harder than you do, physically or in other circumstances. This does not make you better than they, but it should bring you compassion as well as gratitude and thankfulness even in the midst of your struggles.

Chapter 12

Capitol Calling

While I was at Colorado Christian University, I never lived on campus, and until my last year I didn't develop many friendships. Even so, I was blessed through the experiences I had there. Again, in college I didn't date anybody. I had a great desire to, and did attempt to a number of times, but it never worked out. Like in high school, the devil still whispered fears into my head, and I believed many of them.

Though it probably ultimately was less embarrassing than using a walker would have been, the decision to use a wheelchair, may have been part of the reason for my diminished confidence with girls while I was in college. Noticing that there was a segment of people who don't know how to react to a person in a wheelchair, I feared—probably somewhat correctly—that finding any co-eds who were not put-off by a guy using a wheelchair would be hard to do. I feared even more than before that girls would not find me of interest because of my lack of ability to do many of the things others did with ease. I knew better than to believe all of it entirely, but this uncertainty lingered.

As I said above, I had tried to date a few times during college, but to my consternation, when I started to get close, the girl would end up having a serious boyfriend, or fiancée, or just not have much more to do with me. I had many girl *friends*, but not a girlfriend. In my four years in college, knowing and seeing that there were so many quality girls, this is something that hung over me, and it had the potential to leave me with an empty feeling.

Thus, my years of college came to an end. Actually, I had done much better academically in college than high school. While in high school, my grades were mainly mediocre, and I was never in honors anything. At the end of attending CCU, I'd made the Dean's List, was a member of an honors group, and graduated Magna Cum Laude. I suppose that I put more effort into my work! On graduation day I rolled across the stage in my wheelchair to receive my diploma. I said good-bye to the friends I had made and turned to face the "real" world.

After 17 years of continuous schooling, life was completely changing. I had to figure out what to do now, and I wouldn't be seeing my new friends regularly anymore. My thoughts weren't as much about my body—because it hadn't been changing that much, but more on my future outside of school; what would I do?

Thankfully, God had a plan in mind for me. I had a professor, who learned about my interest in, and an aptitude for, politics. He had some contacts at the state capitol and after visiting the Colorado state capitol with a class my senior year, he suggested that I think about becoming a legislator's aide. I didn't have any other goals or aspirations after graduating so I decided to interview. My professor set up the interview and I spoke with the lady in charge of office aides and interns. (The person with whom I spoke is now my friend—Lori Brown.) The interview went well, and she invited me to come back for a second interview. In the meantime, she tried to pair me with a senator who had beliefs and convictions similar to mine. I met with Senator

Scott Renfroe of Greeley. He interviewed me, and soon I had a job as a state senator's aide!

Senator Renfroe and I had similar beliefs, principles, and convictions in basically every area. I admire and look up to him as a leader because, first of all, he is a Christian, and those beliefs permeate every area of his life, but also because he was not a stereo-typical politician. He had principles and stuck to them no matter what, regardless of how popular or unpopular they were. He would not do anything to garner political favor from anyone, and he would invoke Jesus' name on the Senate floor—which at times, evoked much hatred and mocking. Yet he did so without any regrets. He is a model that would be good for all politicians to emulate. During the time that I served as his aide, we became good friends.

Not only was I interested in learning about politics and the legislative process, but I was also interested in seeing how the principles and processes of the United States were implemented. As I wrote earlier, I was a Boy Scout and am an Eagle Scout. A large part of the Scouting program is to educate boys about the United States, its formation, its guiding principles, and civics. Learning these things in Scouts taught me a great appreciation of, and gave me a deep respect for, my nation.

As I went to a private school, I did not learn (as are now taught in the public schools) all the supposed evils of America, but I did learn all about the imperfections of the nation. As I learned all these things however, I learned that my country could be imperfect in many ways, while yet exceptional and good in many other ways. I wasn't necessarily interested much in politics when I was younger, but my dad was always bringing it up at home and my grandparents also probably influenced me some.

I viewed working at the capitol during the legislative session, as a service. Being unable to serve my country militarily, I took great pride in serving as an aide; I considered working for a state legislator a way of serving my country, albeit in a very small way. Serving in government is important, even though I believe the great majority of government positions are a waste and that the government needs to be significantly scaled-down. But...as this isn't a book about politics, I'll move on.

I loved working in the Colorado state capitol. It was a tremendous place to work, with its large open spaces, beautiful architecture, and finely detailed ornamentation. With the Senate Republicans being in the minority, I worked in a large office space filled with cubicles which had a few real offices in the back. Thus, not only was I able to get to know many of the other aides and interns but many of the other senators as well.

The majority party senators mainly had their own individual offices. Being out of school and not really knowing anybody, I quickly made friends at the capitol. I also loved being able to talk about politics on the job! Another benefit which I loved is that my aide name placard gave me access to go on the Senate floor whenever I pleased. I loved to go there when the Senate was in session and watch the proceedings and see the system work.

One morning soon after I first began working there, a man named Dan File introduced himself to me. He invited me to a Bible Study which he led each Tuesday at lunch during the legislative session. This was a pleasant surprise as I didn't know there would be a Christian ministry for staff members at the capitol. It led me to making new friends and became the best time during the session. Life was going well and after working for the first session I was able to go back and work for Senator Renfroe a second session.

Despite being (jokingly) fired nearly three to four times each week, I actually worked for four sessions under Senator Renfroe—his full second and final term in the state Senate. I developed great relationships and friendships during my four years working at the state capitol, and it was a joy to be at work. I loved having a reason to wear a suit and tie every day!

There were senators who, on occasion would kid around with me, and even a senator who occasionally popped me up on two wheels! Perhaps sometimes I spoke with others too much; another senator jokingly claimed that all I did was chat with his aide. Being around such jovial, good-hearted people, and working in that pleasant environment was a delight–the environment in the capitol in general, however, was certainly not all-pleasant! Although I may not have been able to do as much work or stay the long hours like other aides, I am blessed to have been given the opportunity to work there. Not only that, but it was a blessing to have been a witness for Christ through my attitude, speech, and treatment of others during my work.

Truths I've Experienced

Relational Support

> A friend loves at all times, and a brother is born for a time of adversity.
>
> Proverbs 17:17

I have discussed how God uses the hard times of our lives to bring us blessings. Again, the blessings of our trials can be difficult for us to determine, but in my life and dealing with my disorder, I've been consistently blessed by the people around me. When going through a rough patch in life, it's terrific to have people by your side to encourage you through the struggle. Having a family member or a friend who cares for you and cares about what you are facing in life is very uplifting.

I cannot put into words how blessed and grateful I am for all the people who have made a positive impact on my life. Without the support of others, I still could have lived with the struggle with my disorder by God's grace and presence. But doing so would have been much more difficult without the love and support of those whom He has blessed me with and through.

Throughout my life, I've known family members or friends who are facing some sort of predicament but don't want others to know about it, either out of pride or embarrassment. I understand this to a small point, but I find it a wholly foolish train of thought—regardless of one's religious beliefs. My question on this subject is thus: is it better to deal with your problems alone or deal with them with the support and encouragement, and perhaps prayers, of others who care for you? I choose the latter, and the benefits of this have been demonstrated many times in my life! It can be very difficult to overcome a strong sense of pride or embarrassment, but we are relational beings and can deal with difficult circumstances so much better with the love and support of others.

Family serves a huge earthly role in caring for and encouraging individuals in their life struggles. The family unit is integral for this. I am tremendously thankful that I grew up in an intact, strong, and loving household. Even now as an adult, even though my siblings are currently spread out from us geographically, my family unit remains strong. From the time we were kids we have always shared in each other's joys, sadnesses, and hardships. And we continue to do so.

If one of us were to need help with something, we would always help each other. When encouragement or prayer are needed, we are "on it". It has always been so, and this foundation of support gives me and my siblings a strong foundation.

While my family has always been tight knit, certainly, we were not perfect. I'm sure that my siblings and I each have circumstances or missteps that we prefer not to share. But all in all, not much was held back. Sadly, many families are not whole, and many kids lack a great example of how family members can support and encourage one another in a healthy way.

I have been privy to many examples of familial dysfunction at various junctures in my life. Having been raised in the immediate family that that I was, learning the morals I was taught by my parents, and coming to understand Christian principles, I've seen how dysfunction in families can just feed further dysfunction. Especially in the formative years when growing up, kids need good examples, but they also need to know that whenever they face a predicament or dilemma in that life, that they have a parent or a sibling or even extended family member that will listen to them without judgment, encourage, and point them in the right direction. God gave us the family unit I grew up with so that we would learn to love, teach, encourage, and support each other through difficulties, challenges, missteps and tragedies. Yet, sadly in our culture today, the importance of family is being brushed off.

Friendships are also important relationships in life. It can be hard to put into words how extraordinarily blessed I am by friendships in my life. Of course, I don't have many *extremely* close friends, but friends in general, I feel that I do. It is great having friends and others who are not family who genuinely care for you. It is great also to have people you can call upon or go to whenever you are facing trouble.

In life, our individual relationship with Jesus is what ultimately matters, but our relationships with others in this world are extremely important. Being relational is a must if one is to be a disciple of Christ. Life would be wretched if we had nobody to whom we felt close. I don't have a perfect relationship with anybody, and I don't claim to, but relationships are important, and we are instructed in the Bible to build each other up. I've learned, and maybe you have, as well: When facing great adversity, the importance of human support of love, and encouragement, and care is second only to God's support, and the value of such is immeasurable.

Chapter 13

Eyes Opened

After Senator Renfroe was term-limited out of office, I decided not to return to the state capitol. I found myself not doing much of anything for about a year.

My friend Aaron got married in New Hampshire, and at his wedding my former gym teacher, Mrs. Landhuis, told my mom that she thought it would be good to explore the possibility of my having a role at my former school, Denver Christian. So, Mrs. Landhuis spoke to Mrs. Jackson-Gustafson, a counselor at my former school, about seeing if they could utilize my skills in any way. Though I never went to her for counseling, in middle school my friends and I would spend many breaks and lunches in her office, talking to her and eventually doing Bible studies. I was acquainted with Mrs. Jackson-Gustafson in middle school, and over the years since then, she and I became good friends. At some point I was invited to call her by her first name—Jen.

After having returned from Aaron's wedding, Jen reached out to me later that summer. She and I discussed different things I could do as a volunteer at the school. In the fall of 2015, I decided to volunteer twice a week.

It was a blessing to be back and helping at the school which had been such a significant part of my life. And though much had changed, like the location, several staff and teachers from my time were still around.

I served in capacities such as tutoring high school students in one of my favorite high school teacher's classrooms, Mrs. Dyk, working in various elementary classes, and practicing reading with a few first-graders. I was able to speak in a few high school classes about politics and my experience working for the government. I teamed up with the counseling department and spoke with elementary and middle school classes on biblical and character subjects. And I was also able to speak in both an elementary and middle/high school chapel sharing parts of my testimony.

I had a great time there, this second go-around, reconnecting with former teachers and getting to know students of all ages. While it wasn't exactly where I would have chosen to have been at that point in my life, several doors were opened. The first was that I had the ability to travel there. Additionally, the hopeful and gracious response received from people at the school who wanted me to volunteer there was very affirming, and the fact that I loved Denver Christian for the role it played in my life gave me some excitement about serving at the same school that I had attended. Though, in my early 20s, I would have preferred to be working, God showed me this was where I was meant to be.

With my limitations, I'm not able to work a full-time job and make an income to take care of myself. That's one of the biggest struggles I have with my disorder. I want to be self-sufficient, working to take care of myself.

Through this time of volunteering at Denver Christian, I came to a realization. In my circumstances, I have a subtle form of pride. During the period that I was a volunteer at Denver Christian, when asked by others what I did, I found it a bit embarrassing, in essence, to reveal that I volunteered rather than being able to say that I had a job. I felt that volunteering seemed somewhat lazy, that I was relying on others to provide for me while I wasn't supporting myself. Because of my pride, I have always hated the idea of receiving any kind of welfare. For that reason, I have always been careful about how I present myself. I was shocked to discover that though I have major physical issues, I take pride in how I present myself to others—and not only in the area of employment. I will work harder at times when talking to someone to make sure they don't think me slow or less capable because of my appearance or voice. I take pride in presenting myself so that any person who sees me will perceive me to be as capable as I am. I suppose that this pride stems from the fear of being perceived as less than what and who I am.

Rather than being wholly proud of who God made me and the life He has given me, many times I have given in to seeing myself through the eyes of others. Specifically, I have given in to seeing myself through the eyes of those who only see my wheelchair and body, who see only what I am unable to do. This leaves me feeling inferior to them because of my inabilities.

I certainly cannot say that I have conquered this form of pride, but my eyes have been opened to it. Who I am as a person won't change in many ways, and there are many parts of me, notably physically, that I cannot change. I cannot live according to how I think others perceive me. Rather, I must live my life in the best way I can. I also have to be thankful for the opportunities that have been given to me, even when I desired employment and instead had the opportunity to volunteer.

Though I still desired employment, I was pleased that, the following school year, God again gave me the opportunity to return to Denver Christian, and I looked forward to what God had in store for me the next school year!

Truths I've Experienced

Adversity

> I have told you these things, so that in me you may have peace. In this world you will have trouble. But take heart! I have overcome the world.
>
> John 16:33

Adversity—though certainly not welcomed with open arms—is a sure part of life and a huge determining factor in the development of our character. While this is true for all people, for Christians, adversity can have an even heavier impact: it can also affect beliefs. Hardships greatly shape our relationship with God, these can make or break a Christian's faith. For unbelievers, it can lead one towards God or completely embitter one against the thought of God. While, in themselves, times of trial are terrible, the resulting outcomes of such seasons in our lives can be equally bad or even worse. That is why it is so important to find something good in hardships. With the right attitude, such seasons can also lead to great growth in our life.

Again, my physical disorder is not the sole adversity I face in my life, but it i1s one of the most prominent. When I ponder my life—my circumstances, my difficulties, my sins, my relationships, my blessings, how my Lord has walked with me—I can plainly see that though I have faced much adversity, the good in my life far outweighs the bad. I have come to see that my disorder is ultimately a blessing because of the work that God enables me to do through it. I most definitely become frustrated with my circumstances at many times, but in the grand scheme of things, knowing how my trials have shaped my character and faith as well as how they have given me unique opportunities to serve: it has been worth it.

Adversity is one of my favorite subjects to talk about. This is not because I know everything about the subject or even understand God's ultimate purpose for it. I certainly don't! But because of my life-circumstances, I am able to relate much more with, and speak into the lives of, others. I've seen the different ways people deal with trial; some persevere and come out better from it, and some simply give in and allow the darkness to overcome them. I developed this above concept concerning trials while I was in high school, and it seemed original to me at the time, though now I know that others have also explored it.

This next part explains my understanding about the choice a Christian must make when responding to adversity. The choice available to the Christian heart is a simple juxtaposition. In times of trial or distress, a Christian can either run towards God and become stronger in faith or forsake God and fall into bitterness. Though I came to this idea when I was young, I still hold this to be true, having witnessed it in others as well as first-hand.

Going back again to John 16:33, Jesus tells us "In this world you will have trouble. But take heart! I have overcome the world." We will all face trouble in our lifetimes—some more than others—but trouble itself is an equal opportunity guarantee. The question for the Christian experiencing adversity is whether or not he or she will trust these words of Jesus and place hope and trust in Him when experiencing the hardship.

Throughout my years dealing with my physical situation, I have chosen to run to God. My trust in Him, though not perfect, has greatly strengthened my faith and allowed me to view my disorder as a blessing rather than as a detriment. With my physical troubles, I honestly never directed anger towards God. This doesn't make me righteous or indicate that I deal with things better than other Christians.

In fact, I have gone through periods of my life during which I felt that I may be handling things incorrectly because I wasn't wrestling with God over this. It probably started in high school, but especially when I got into college; theology classes and chapels proclaimed that being mad at God because of certain things that happen to us is normal and healthy. On top of that, doubting God is also something everybody goes through, and that is normal and can strengthen faith.

Since I didn't harbor anger or frustration towards God because of my body, I began to truly question whether or not I had been too laid-back or apathetic in my relationship with God. This seemed a possibility as I had not gone through such struggles as most other people seemed to. I wondered if my faith was not developing and strengthening because of the absence of these conflicts. To this day, I cannot recall a time during which I have harbored anger against the Lord for my circumstances, or doubted His existence and or His role in my life.

As I have said, of course I get angry and frustrated many times in my life when my body fails me, when I'm limited because I physically cannot do something. In those times I do plead to the Lord for healing, for mercy on my body. Yet in those moments when my ire can rise, I realize, sometimes to my selfish dismay, that the Lord has been faithful in my life. God has plans for me, even though they may not take the form that I would like. He is with me in those difficult moments and will be with me throughout my future. Furthermore, it would only harm me if I were to hold a grudge against Him

As far as doubting, I've still not (and hope never to) hit a point of that in my life. Like other Christians, my relationship with God throughout life has had fluctuations. I have periods in my life where I feel very close to God and am on fire for Him. And conversely, and the blame for this is mine, I have lulls in my life where I become distracted by sin and distance myself from God. In those lulls, it can be easy to feel that God isn't close. And I think this is a common misconception many Christians fall into at times. God is always close. But we sometimes distance ourselves through sin, or distraction, or mis-ordered priorities, and it can be harder to be attuned to God.

In the fluctuations of my faith, I've always clung to God. As my faith has matured (and that is a lifelong process), I have come to understand that every Christian's faith is different. God deals with each of us differently. Some people doubt, some may not. Some rage at God, some do not. Growing up, I have met other people who have not doubted or been angry at God over their trials. It simply differs for each person, and can depend on the situations encountered. Not doubting or holding anger against God is fine; doubting or being angry at God is fine as well. Either of these responses, as long as they do not lead a person out of their faith, are good and normal. They have the potential to further strengthen faith.

These extremes that I just mentioned can play a large role in determining whether a person who is facing difficult circumstances will seek or reject God. Though in my life I have not gone in the direction of abandoning God in hardship, I have been a witness to people who have done this. The great thing about these possible reactions to difficulties, is that they do not apply only to Christians. Times of trial affect every person deeply, whether or not the person believes in God. Circumstances can lead Christians or unbelievers toward God or away from Him.

I have seen many examples of various responses to hardship. I have seen Christians with weak faith, Christians with strong faith, as well as unbelievers who assert they don't believe in Jesus. Whichever group one falls into, almost every person alive can face a trial so great that it can overcome them.

Some Christians may feel abandonment, thinking that because they are a believer, that God will shield them from terrible hardship. Or some may immediately expect God's intervention and help. Still others may feel rejection, as they don't perceive that God is helping as much as they would like. Christians might also simply get caught up in the trial and take their focus off of God. Unbelievers may reject God, simply saying that if a loving God exists, He wouldn't allow such horrible things to happen in life.

I have also heard from some people that God can't relate to their circumstances or sufferings. "Jesus didn't deal with what I'm going through, so He can't empathize." The original ancient Greek that the New Testament was written in, records 12 instances in the Gospels where a particular word for "compassion" is used. These instances include when Jesus had compassion for those who had physical maladies, for the multitudes or crowds and their plights and misdirection, as well as in a few parables. The Greek word is rendered in English as *splagchnizomai*: it means, "to have the bowels yearn that is (figuratively), feel sympathy to pity: – have (be moved with) compassion."[1]

This amazing insight displays to me in my circumstances, that the Almighty God has so much love for a mere mortal like me, but it goes beyond that; He knows what I live with and He has sorrow knowing what I personally deal with. God hurts with me!

This goes even further. Not only is God concerned about his followers' physical hardships, but by the maladies of unbelievers as well. God is not simply distressed by the physical trials people face, but by the other plights in life that we face as well. And in addition to God's concern about our trials, He is distressed about those who do not know or believe in Him. Wherever you are in life, whether you believe in God or not, we all face trouble. The difficulty may be physical, emotional, financial, or, come in some other form. God knows what you face personally and He loves you so much that your hardships distress God to figurative discomfort. God hurts with you! This tremendous insight into God's love shows that God isn't just sitting in Heaven watching our life, stoically ignoring our personal problems. He physically aches *with* us.

No matter who you are, and despite your feelings about God's action or empathy, you have options in a time of trial. The choice to reject God and to try to persevere through the struggle without Him exists, and choosing that option will lead to a long and terribly arduous process. I've not been down this road, but I have seen that often its outcome is bitterness, anger, and self–pity. When one takes this path, the end of that road is further trouble and sorrow mounting on top of hardship.

The other path I see in times of trial is turning to God. Again, consider younger Christians, stronger Christians, and unbelievers. If you face a difficult trial and choose to trust in God, His Word promises that you will be given both comfort and strength to persevere. This does not mean that the process will be easy. Nor does it mean that the suffering will quickly go away.

It does mean, however, that there will be hope. There is hope in the God who loves you and who promises to help and to comfort you. There is hope in that despite trials, God will make you stronger and that you have another life to look forward to that is free from suffering. God will take away all their tears. There will be no more death or sorrow or crying or pain. All the old things have passed away (Revelation 21:4). Also remember that in Romans 8:28, we are told that adversities will be used for good and may pave the way for more opportunities to serve God and others in the future. Both the weak and the strong Christian, when turned to God, will grow stronger in faith. When in trouble, if the unbeliever takes a chance and turns to God, faith may be found.

I see two choices with contrary outcomes: one with a good, and the other a bad. One, which despite hardship, leads to strength, and one which succumbs to hardship and leads to self-destruction. We have a God who loves us so greatly that He has promised not to leave us, but to be our help in all areas of our lives.

Chapter 14

Difficult Realities

In the fall of 2016, I again returned to Denver Christian for my second school year to volunteer. This year, my focus was going to be more on helping in both of the preschool classes. I had a lot of fun being around and playing with those kids. For a portion of the day, I was also assigned as a para-educator to a middle-school student to offer support during some classes as well as with assignments. I enjoyed working and talking with this student. The year was going great, and I was very excited to go to work during the week.

In late October of that year, my parents and I took a trip to the Cayman Islands. I am not a beach person, but it was very nice there and I had a good time. However, I was pretty tired the whole week; I fell asleep numerous times on the beach with my head up while sitting upright in my chair! I assumed it was because the couch bed that I was sleeping in made my back sore.

I had a doctor's appointment a few days after we returned home. There I learned that my heart rate had quickened; the AFib had returned. I called my cardiologist, and he recommended that I start a medicine called Amiodarone which would help my heart to both slow down and to maintain a better rhythm. This medicine, however, takes several days to build up in the body and start working. I began this medication on a Friday, without having had any communication with *my* doctors over the weekend. My dad was gone that weekend because right after vacation, he had taken another week off to go elk hunting! Consequently, only my mom and I were at home for the weekend and the following week.

I could not really tell if the medicine was doing much of anything over the weekend, but I felt better mentally being on it. I was still feeling very tired though and hoped that I would get some rest before going back to the school that week. I went to sleep that Sunday and woke up in the middle of the night, technically very early Monday morning. It is not unusual for me to wake up in the middle of the night. Many times, I have nightmares—usually about falling down the stairs! I don't know what causes those, but some of that may be due to all the medicine I take.

Anyways, this was different. When I woke up, my heart was very uncomfortable and felt like it was straining. My breathing was also off. When I took a deep breath, I was unable to fully inhale; my body would allow me to breathe in only so much. I called for my mom, and somehow knowing it wasn't just a nightmare, she immediately ran to my room. We decided to head to the emergency room, not calling for an ambulance because things didn't seem dire, and we didn't live that close to a hospital. So, I got up, dressed, ascended the stairs using the stair lift, and left the house.

The sky was beautiful that night, and as we were getting into the car, I could see so many stars. I took a moment to look at them, but my mom, worried, told me to get in the car! The 25-minute trip from my house to the University of Colorado Hospital was uneventful. My mom gave my dad a call and told him I was going to the hospital, so my dad left Steamboat Springs where he was hunting, to come back down to Aurora

Difficult Realities

where I would be. I arrived and got checked in, and my symptoms hadn't changed.

While waiting in my bay in the ER, my Aunt Dee Dee and soon to be uncle Ed came to see me. We visited until my dad returned from the mountains—a four-hour trip. After having an EKG, blood tests, and speaking with doctors, we learned that the strain and discomfort were due to my AFib (my heart not having responded to the new medicine yet) and that my not being able to breathe deeply was because my AFib had caused blood to enter into one of my lungs.

My aunt and Ed left, and soon after their departure, things started to go downhill. The nurse had given me an antibiotic for some reason, and it really started to affect my processing. As I looked around, I literally saw stars or dots everywhere my eyes moved.

That started to subside and suddenly my blood pressure started to dive. The nurses were searching for a number of minutes for my pulse, but they were unsuccessful. I can't say what it was like in the room because I was not in my senses, but I think a lot of those machines got really noisy. My parents were still in the room, and I briefly remember their fear and anxiety in those moments.

With my blood pressure descending, I became very sleepy. I wasn't even worried; I just wanted to close my eyes. I remember at one point a doctor saying to me, "Stay with me, David!" It's kind of a blur but, somehow, I regained some awareness and knew that they were working on putting an emergency line down the carotid artery from my neck to my heart. This way, any medicine they gave me would work instantly. They were able to find a medicine that worked to bring my blood pressure back to normal and lower my heart rate.

I feel badly for my parents and what they had to witness and go through in that situation, because things did not look good for me. After being stabilized, I was transferred to the ICU. I didn't even have the desire to think about the events that had transpired, I just wanted to sleep.

At some point after I went into the ICU that same morning, there was another little scare. I had an Echocardiogram (Echo)—a sonogram to see inside the heart, and the cardiologist told me that a blood clot was found. That is not something anyone wants to hear, because a blood clot can lead to more troubles. Well, time—filled with various consultations of which I recall little, and definitely some praying—went by.

That afternoon or so, the attending doctors ordered another Echo. (Again, all the events during the first day were a bit hazy for me). They performed the Echo again and were unable to find the blood clot. I believe God took that clot away, and thankfully, I did not have to deal with the issues a blood clot could lead to on top of everything else.

Word about my hospitalization spread among my family and friends, and not long after I had learned the news of the clot having disappeared and my condition stabilizing, I began to have many visitors. Family who lived in town came by, as well as a number of friends. As I've said, I appreciate nurses, and I had a very skilled one at the hospital I was staying in. Eventually, Jeanelle and Josh—my brother-in-law, and Daniel were able to fly in. Hope, my sister-in-law, had to stay in Oklahoma, to take care of my nieces—Grace and Julia.

It was good to have my parents and all these other dear ones around most of the time, even though I still slept often. I even fell asleep on election night, and I was hoping to watch some results for the presidency! I wasn't too worried about missing it though, as I had a feeling about how it would turn out.

It seemed I had dodged the bullet of the hated catheter in this hospital episode. But then one day a nurse grew worried about my urine output. I was somewhat dehydrated when I arrived at the hospital and had not been drinking much (other than the fluids I was getting through the IV) so the times when I had to pee were few and far between. He threatened me with a catheter if I couldn't go, so I tried and tried but could not.

I don't deal well with being under pressure; peeing on demand wasn't going to work! So, despite my protests, I got the blasted catheter inserted, awake no less, and the thing was uncomfortable. After having it for a pretty short time, the nurses decided to remove it, and what do you know—my system functioned fine. I did not and still don't think the catheter was necessary though; if I'd had time to try to go at my own pace, I probably would have!

After being at University Hospital for three or four days, my doctors wanted me transferred to St. Joseph's, a hospital run by my insurance provider. This hospital has access to all my medical records. I travelled in style: for the first time in my life, I got an ambulance ride! When I arrived at St. Joseph's, I went up to my new room in the ICU and there met my nurse, Melissa. As she was helping me transfer beds and hooking me up to the machines in the room, she somehow sprayed me almost up my nose with saline. We both laughed about it, and from that moment, I knew I would like her.

Over the course of my time at St. Joseph's, Melissa was a terrific nurse. She had a great sense of humor, was very caring and compassionate, and quite often went beyond her duties helping me. She even gave me a sponge bath one day, even though that is the Certified Nursing Assistant's job. I've seen a number of nurses in my days, but she is the one I will certainly always remember, and I am very thankful that God blessed me with her at that time.

Even after transferring to St. Joseph's Hospital, I was blessed again to have many visitors! My family members were still in town, and they made the move between hospitals as my parents did. In addition to visits from family and friends, I was also paid a visit by my electrophysiology cardiologist, Dr. Lewkowiez.

The main thing we discussed was when the time may come to take a different approach to address my heart rhythms. The doctor explained that over time, as my heart rhythms continued to decline, a procedure called an ablation might be helpful. An ablation is where a patient is put under anesthesia and the surgeon goes up an artery with a tool to burn certain electrical circuits around the heart to re-wire it. He had never done this procedure on somebody with Friedreich's, and at that time, there wasn't information about anybody with this disorder having had the procedure. Given the lack of information, Dr. Lewkowiez wasn't even sure if my heart circuits would be in good enough shape for the ablation. This was something he would not be able to assess until actually going in and seeing my heart.

I was hoping not to undergo more surgeries, so I hoped I would not need to exercise this option. The doctor had more to discuss, but my room was pretty busy, so he said he would come back later.

Eventually, my brother, and my sister and her husband, had to get back home after spending four or five days with me, so things got a little quieter in the room. I was very thankful that they had come to spend time with me during this crisis, but at the same time, I expected nothing less. They have always come through for me.

Unfortunately, there wasn't anything I could do in the hospital to earn a speedier release. My cardio situation paired with my immobility, pretty much just allowed me to lie in the bed. That became frustrating, because I felt so stuck and weak simply doing nothing.

Since that night in the ER, however, whatever medicine I had been given was working. My heart had stabilized. I actually didn't get too bored either, mostly because I always had people with whom I could talk. Thankfully, after five days in the ICU, I was transferred out. Although I was glad to be leaving the ICU, I was sad that I would no longer see Melissa.

When transferred to the regular Cardiac Unit, I ended up having a brash New Yorker as a nurse during the day. I still had the line in my neck that was inserted during my time in the ER five days before, and asked him how long it might be before that could be removed. He said that it would probably be within the next few days, because they worry about patients contracting infections in hospitals. "Infections are the leading killer of people at hospitals," he said. That was some terrific bedside manner! He wasn't my favorite nurse!

I did have another interesting encounter with a nurse whom I did appreciate. One of the night nurses had seen my mom in the hallway and had noticed the cross on her neck. She asked if my mom was a Christian and if it would be okay if the three of us could pray together for me. This nurse, who was Catholic, prayed for me in my hospital room. She even had holy water from somewhere in France. I appreciated this kind and generous consideration, as I never had a staff member at the hospital leading a prayer for me. However, that nurse and the experience of praying together was another way of God showing me His presence.

Even after moving from the ICU, again I was fortunate to see many people. One night, I had around 15 people visiting me, at the same time! Having visitors is always an integral part of recovery in the hospital. Chatting with loved ones is invariably rejuvenating, and was especially so in this situation. Receiving their care and compassion was very comforting and encouraging. And it made the time go by faster.

Over the duration of my hospitalization, I had a number of visitors from a number of places. I had people visit from their various locales in Colorado. My friend Dan File came from the mountains. An uncle flew in from Texas, and a cousin from Indiana. My siblings from out-of-state had already visited. And this list does not include those who were praying for me—and I don't know if I could even count all of them! I figured I had prayers from Hawaii all the way across the country to Virginia! I was in good hands!

I was becoming more and more eager to go home after a week since this entire ordeal had started. At that point, the worst was behind me, and I simply wanted to move forward. I believe it was on my final day in the hospital, that I met again with Dr. Lewkowiez to discuss what lay ahead.

My parents and I weren't sure what to expect as we'd never had to face the hard realities of my heart situation before this experience. Doctor Lewkowiez was very blunt and straightforward with the information, explaining everything. He said that I would need to remain on a heart medication. The Amiodarone was working very, very well, but the longer a person remains on it, the greater the chance of several nasty side effects. There was also the option of trying a different medication which, while also being very effective, was not quite as effective as Amiodarone. But, in its favor, this other medicine had fewer side effects. Those were pretty much my two medication options for stabilizing my heart rhythm.

Then came the more difficult portion of the conversation. My heart troubles would continually worsen over time, so the doctor told me about more that could be done in the future besides medication. The ablation which he had talked about earlier was one choice. A pacemaker was another option. A third—and the least desirable option in my mind—was a defibrillator.

A defibrillator sounded awful because it would be surgically placed onto my heart. Then, it would deliver a very painful, but lifesaving, shock whenever it sends the heart going out of rhythm. A defibrillator shock could add more years to my life. However, there was a downside. As someone with a defibrillator draws near to death, the dying process can be long and extremely painful. As the heart starts to fail and wants to quit, the defibrillator, realizing that the heart continues to go out of rhythm, starts to continually shock the heart and revive the person. In essence, it sounds like it can be a painful and drawn-out death.

Hearing these things scared me. The doctor said that we didn't know how long it would take for my condition to require the necessity of making a choice. Part of the reason for this uncertainty is because of my disorder and its degenerative nature. He said that, overall, I probably wouldn't be looking at more than a decade, relatively, of life, based on my disorder compounded with my heart troubles.

I knew that my life expectancy must be lower because of my condition and that at some point in the future I would have to contemplate these life and death matters. But at that point in my life, it was a terribly harsh reality that I was facing. I was very upset after that conversation because, as for everybody, facing the reality of death is terrifying!

I was only 27 years old, and there was still much I wanted to do in my life. I told my mom that even so, I believed my life was in the Lord's hands. There was nothing I could do to change the situation. The doctor apologized to my dad because things had gotten emotional, but my dad told him we appreciated his frankness.

With all these thoughts swirling in my head after that conversation that morning, I was thankful I was going to be leaving the hospital that day. I finally got to have every needle, tube, and hose that had been poked into me removed, and that was a relief. However, the line being pulled from my neck was a strange feeling!

I had been in the hospital a full week, the longest time I had been stuck in one. With great joy, my parents and I finally headed home!

It was so good, and restful, to be back home. It was very nice not to be interrupted while sleeping! The reality that I had been so close to dying had been in my mind all along, but it didn't really sink in until after I had returned from the hospital and things began to calm down. Now, I had more time to think about it. It surprised me, but the first few nights back I somewhat dreaded going to sleep in my own bed.

Though it was good to be in my bed, I experienced a degree of PTSD, because it was in this bed that I had woken up when the situation started to go downhill. I was a bit leery, wondering if the same things would happen again. I feared that, while alone in my bed, I might again feel my heart acting strangely.

It took many weeks for my body to recover from everything it had gone through and from having laid in the hospital bed for a week.

At times I wanted to keep myself busy at home, but so often I did not have the motivation to do much! Thinking about death made me uneasy, especially initially after my time in the hospital. I couldn't sit back anymore knowing that my health and body would progressively deteriorate. I had always known that this reality was in my future, but I thought, *things are still good right now and I don't need to dwell on it.* Yet, that time was now upon me; I couldn't ignore it anymore.

I still had faith in God and hope for the future, but my humanity caused me to fear for my physical flesh and blood. I remember my Uncle John relaying to me while I was in the hospital that Jesus was afraid of dying before going to the cross. "The spirit is willing, but the flesh is weak (Matthew 26:41)." It was okay to be a Christian and still fear dying, even knowing that my future is an eternity in heaven. That fear is just part of being human. I am grateful that my Uncle John shared these thoughts with me.

I had to wait until January to return to Denver Christian. It was great to see all the other teachers, but probably even better to be spending time with all those children again. I finished that school year and even applied for a pre-school teaching job for the next year. That was my last year volunteering at Denver Christian. In the years volunteering there, I have been able to reconnect with some of my old teachers and become friends with others as well as develop relationships with many students. I was very blessed by my time there.

One of the most treasured things that came from my experience volunteering at Denver Christian was when Mrs. Dyk gave me a card which she explained was from an anonymous student. The card told me how this person admired me and how, as I moved about through the school, they could see Jesus through my joy, attitude, and strength. I read the card and was very touched by it. This note wasn't a boost to my ego, but rather an encouragement for me on a much deeper level. God was showing me my purpose for being at Denver Christian at that time and was assuring me that He was working through me. That is what I wanted: to be Christ's witness through my life. That I have been His witness has been confirmed to me from others before, but it was touching to hear it from a high schooler.

Partly because I did not get hired for the pre-school job, and partly because I was ready to move on to something else, I decided that I would not return to DC the following year. I didn't know what or where I would be in the future, but I would find out. It turned out that the next year I ended up mostly being at home. Of course, I did go and see friends and family when I could.

Each Friday I joined my grandparents, and eventually also my Aunt Dee Dee, as we all volunteered at the Alzheimer's Center. This is something in which I had been participating with my Grandma and Grandpa Car since I was in middle school.

I started going as a service project for Boy Scouts, and joined my grandparents as they read the Bible and sang hymns with the residents every Friday afternoon. Almost two decades later, I still do this with my grandpa and aunt, and over the past seven years or so, afterwards some of my family and friends have gone to "happy hour" somewhere and use it as a time to connect with each other!

I also did not merely twiddle my thumbs while I was at home; I had projects to do. Since working at the capitol and especially since working at Denver Christian, I knew that physically, working wasn't really going to be an option for me, even though I would have liked to work. Being home however, kept the schedule open for my parents and me to be able to go on trips. I enjoy traveling and having the opportunity to go and see different places in my state, the country, and the world. If I were able, this is something that I could do all the time. I enjoyed travels and being at home, but I knew that God wanted me somewhere and doing more than just being at home; I would never have guessed, however, where He was leading me.

Truths I've Experienced

Hope

There are also heavenly bodies and there are earthly bodies; but the splendor of the heavenly bodies is one kind, and the splendor of the earthly bodies is another. So it will be with the resurrection of the dead. The body that is sown is perishable, it is raised imperishable; it is sown in dishonor, it is raised in glory; it is sown in weakness, it is raised in power; it is sown a natural body, it is raised a spiritual body. If there is a natural body, there is also a spiritual body. And just as we have borne the image of the earthly man, so shall we bear the image of the heavenly man. For the perishable must clothe itself with the imperishable, and the mortal with immortality. When the perishable has been clothed with the imperishable and the mortal with immortality, then the saying that is written will come true, "Death has been swallowed up in victory."

Excerpted from 1:40-54

I've mentioned this briefly, but now I would like to talk about one of my favorite themes: hope in death. Hope is a driving factor in my life, as it is in all Christians' lives. Even for people who do not believe in Jesus as their savior, hope plays a large role in everyday life. Hope is desire, excitement, longing for, looking forward to something. It may be something as simple as a meal, a class, something at work, or an outing to look forward to which could make the ordinary day better because something good is coming.

Hope also comes in more notable ways: school or job opportunities, dates or weddings, vacations, material things we get to tinker around with. Yet as hope plays an important part in the life of each person, Christian hope, ultimately, is very different.

Christians are not solely looking to hope in this life, but mainly in the next. We are promised forgiveness of all our wrongs done in life as soon as we repent and believe in Jesus Christ as Savior. Better yet, when we die, we get to spend our eternal life in heaven, in perfection, with our loving God; and not having to suffer the consequences of Hell because of our unrepentant sin. What great hope is this to get us through the dredges of life! What better reason to go through trials and hardships in this life knowing that our situation will get infinitely better when we die!

My hope of eternal life, living in perfection with Christ Almighty who loves me, and whom I love, is the greatest and ultimate hope that I have. What better than eternal love, life, and perfection to look forward to amid life's great discouragements and numerous imperfections! As this is my hope, it also drives me to share my testimony: what God has done for me, to share the Gospel—the good news and truth, with those who do not know it. Alongside many others, I have more hope because of my faith. As I have said, my only hope for physical improvement is because I have a relationship with the One who is able to bring that—the One who created me.

Greater than the hope of being healed in this life is the next hope: upon resurrection from death, believers will be accepted into Heaven, which comes with yet another great promise. For the rest of eternity—for forever—Christians get new bodies! Paul writes extensively about this in 1 Corinthians 15 (quoted at the beginning of this section).

That passage provides a great message of hope in death, and of assurance in serving the Lord. This passage excites me, because it gives me a small glimpse of what I have to look forward to. I'm living in a very broken body day by day, and the promise of a new one is beyond compare. That when I die, I will have a new body that will become imperishable and immortal and turn from weakness to strength is a promise, I can hardly imagine. I don't know exactly what all my heavenly body will be or look like, but I believe that it will be my body restored and improved; I can't wait!

Again, I want to clarify to the readers and hearers of my story and faith. Simply put, I did not choose to become a Christian solely because of my body and life circumstances. (In fact, I was a Christian before I knew of my having Friedreich's Ataxia.) I am not a Christian just because of the eternal promise of a new, restored, and perfect body. I am not a Christian to simply cling to a belief that I may be healed. I am not a Christian solely because of how I have had to live with my body and for how the Lord has helped me with my struggles through the years. Those are all perks. I am a Christian because I am assured salvation through the blood of Jesus and will be spending eternity with God, in His presence.

As I wrote before, my faith is based on God's grace and His love for me. I like to imagine, every now and then, my life without God. I consider of the "what if" scenario had I rejected God.

In this "what if" scenario in my mind, I could have turned that anger against God and decided that God is non-existent because if a loving and all-powerful God such as I had learned about in school and church existed, He surely would not allow something like this to happen. Upon diagnosis in seventh grade, it could have been terribly easy for me to fall into despair and anger knowing that I had a normal body and learning that in the coming years it would fall apart causing my life to change dramatically. I still would have had spinal fusion surgery, but rather than clinging to faith, I would only have capitulated to more pain, misery, and bitterness.

In this alternate-path thought experiment, as I went through high school, watching my body slowly fail year after year, and eventually losing my independence bit by bit, life could only have gotten worse. My self-pity would have increased greatly. Beginning college when I had recently begun using a wheelchair, and having completely lost the ability to walk, I could have held a tremendous pity party. Later, finding out about my heart, finding out about my sleep problems, slowly seeing my muscles weaken further, my bitterness could surely have grown.

If I had fallen into this period of self-pity, and loathing of the very life I had been given, I don't know if I would have the friends I have. I would probably be a horribly grumpy person—one whom people would not really want much to do with. I believe that I would have been depressed, discouraged, hopeless, and bitter. What would I have to be joyful about, or to look forward to if I believed that I am stuck in this predicament for life, and when life ends it ends?

Many times, I have thought about what my life would have been without God, and sometimes if I think about it too long, those thoughts scare me! I was given guidance by family, friends, the church, my school, and the Lord sought me. Far from wishing that I never would have had this disorder, I'm thankful for it and for how it is changed my life and strengthened my faith.

I surmise that if I were not disabled, I would not be in a better place than I am. It can be hard for some around me, my parents especially, to understand why my disorder is a good thing and why I believe it's a good thing, and that God's greatest blessings come out of this tribulation.

To be clear, while I am thankful for my disorder and how it has changed my life for the better in many ways, I do have many desires contrary to it as well. I am human and there are numerous times when I become terribly frustrated with my body. I absolutely hate that if I fall out of my chair, I can't get back up on my own. I hate having to rely on others all the time to be driven somewhere. I hate not being able to wake up and get out of bed independently. I hate that using the restroom is always a chore. I hate that I can't go up or down a staircase. I hate that I can't reach items on shelves. These are a tiny fraction of the amount of things that I get frustrated about as I live within the limits of my disorder. I can get terribly frustrated at my circumstances, and I continually pray that God would heal me in this lifetime.

All that said, my hope is both in what could be in this life and in what certainly will be in the next. Being physically healed would be tremendous—an amazing miracle—and I greatly desire that, but it is not the endgame in my life. A final verse which, if believed, offers great encouragement to those dealing with suffering in this life and promising hope for the next, comes from 2 Corinthians 4:17, "For our light and momentary troubles are achieving for us an eternal glory that far outweighs them all." This can be an easy verse to glance over without really considering it in the busyness of our lives. But it holds great meaning.

When I read this verse, I see my troubles from Friedreich's Ataxia are described as "light and momentary". The impact of this disorder on my life is significant and has been significant from even before the time of my diagnosis (as that is why my parents were concerned enough to look into this). I am very limited from doing many of the things I wish to because of it. It has greatly changed my life and will continue to do so as long as I live. Friedreich's Ataxia is not really a "light trouble". And "momentary"? Certainly not, because I have lived with it constantly, so it's not that, either.

Everybody has troubles—whether they be physical, mental, emotional, financial, relational, etc, etc. Our troubles may last hours weeks, months, or years! They certainly do not seem light or momentary to us. Yet, when I slow down and think about this verse more deeply, my thoughts differ greatly.

Initially, no, it does not seem that my daily troubles with my body are light or momentary. Yet when I see that my sufferings are being used to glorify and serve God, I am humbled. I am achieving an eternal glory in Heaven with Christ—who unfathomably loves me! I am promised the glories of eternal life and perfection—the glory of having a perfect, restored heavenly body, as well as being sinless! Most importantly I will live in the glory of being in God's presence— and have, even here on this earth, experienced that to a degree! Then ultimately, yes, this does far outweigh any and all of my sufferings in this life! And when I focus on that second part of the verse then, in the grand scope of things, compared to eternal life my troubles here are *very* momentary. Eternity is forever, our years in this life are but a blip. What an amazing promise this is!

Chapter 15

Voluntarily Visiting the Hospital

Jumping to the fall of 2017, I was still taking Amiodarone, the medicine with all the side effects. As mentioned before, Dr. Lewkowiez suggested I try a different heart rate medication called Tikosyn, the alternative medication which I had heard about in the hospital one year prior. I was cautioned that the body has to decide whether or not it will accept this medication. If my body accepted this medication, I would have a temporary reprieve from the Amiodarone and its side effects. To see if it was possible to switch, I would have to stay at the hospital over a weekend. Nothing was wrong that necessitated my stay, but if my body rejected the medicine, it would have been life-threatening. Thus, it was necessary for me to be monitored.

Though not terribly excited to be hanging around in the bed in the hospital, I went. I was hoping this medicine would have allowed me more medication options down the road with my heart problems. However, it did not go that way.

Even though I was never physically uncomfortable, it was somehow clear to the medical staff that my heart was not reacting well to the new medicine. The doctor told me that the Tikosyn wasn't going to be an option; my body didn't like it.

This was disheartening because my medical options suddenly lessened. The only medication that I could take for my heart now was Amiodarone. Thankfully though, apart from learning that, nothing much was changing with my heart.

Though nothing had changed with the situation with my heart, near the end of 2017, I decided that I really needed to change what I was doing during the week. I started looking for something else to do, somewhere new to volunteer. It took a long time to pray, research, and think about where I might be interested in volunteering. But in time I came upon a possibility that stuck in my head.

I couldn't believe it, but I was looking at Children's Hospital Colorado! I'm sure that it was God putting this on my heart and in my mind, because ever since I was a kid in the hospital, I had decided that I wanted nothing to do with working for, or even being at, Children's Hospital.

As a youngster, it was just terribly sad to see all these kids, many of them younger than I, having to deal with horrible things like disabilities and cancer. Yet God worked through my experiences. I contacted a friend named Sarah Scott who worked at Children's Hospital.

I asked Sarah about the different things volunteers at the hospital did and if there was anything I would be capable of doing. After conversing, more prayer, and thought, I applied for an interview to become a volunteer.

I had read that the process of becoming a volunteer could take a number of weeks or even months, so I was surprised to be contacted relatively quickly about an interview. Sarah had helped the process along and had also spoken about me with the volunteer coordinator. She did so much that when I came in, it was

Voluntarily Visiting the Hospital

hardly an interview! So, the following spring I became a volunteer at Children's Hospital.

It was agreed upon that I would help out in what was called the Creative Play Center; this was pretty much the daycare/play area for siblings–of–patients. The age requirements for those who attended this daycare ranged in age from babies to a maximum age of ten years. The Creative Play Center was usually populated with kids, occasionally another volunteer or two, me, and the staff member in charge.

The staff member who was in charge was named Barbara, and she became a great friend of mine. We got to know each other pretty well because at first it was very slow in that room. No kids came during the three hours that I was there, so we just chatted the whole time. Eventually some days some kids started to come, and some days many came! Since I had worked in the preschool at Denver Christian not long before, I greatly enjoyed my time here! Most of the kids who were dropped off ranged in age from babies to six-year-olds and I really enjoyed seeing so many young kids! It was fun; I was able to just hang out with, play with, and talk with these kids.

The kids were as curious as any kids are with me, wanting to know what happened to me, or about what I do at home, or wanting to push me or sit on my lap. I volunteered in that room for three hours twice a week for almost two years.

One day I let a rambunctious and fun boy push me around in my wheelchair. He suddenly—though, I am certain unintentionally—pushed me into a wall. This snapped the blasted brake from the side of my wheelchair! It wasn't a big deal however, and otherwise everything was fine.

My time volunteering in the Creative Play Center also turned out to be a blessing because in order to take the bus to the hospital I had to go into town. So my mom dropped me off at my Grandpa Car's house where the bus would pick me up. I was able to have between 30 minutes to an hour with my grandpa in the morning, and then a number of hours in the afternoon when I returned before my dad picked me up to go back home.

By the summer of 2019, Barbara was leaving her position and I also wanted a change. Although I sincerely enjoyed my time with the little kids, I wanted to be around kids who were actually *in* the hospital. That was much of the reason I wanted to volunteer there in the first place. So, I spoke again with Sarah, and, mainly because of her efforts, I had the opportunity to move to the Tween Zone.

The Tween Zone was a place at the hospital where teenagers can go and lounge. It had 3-D printers, crafts, video games, a theater, a pool table, and more. Many of the teenagers who dropped in were siblings of patients, but as I had hoped, patients were also allowed. So, I started to work there and enjoyed the company of the older kids. Many times, I spoke with and interacted with kids while they were playing video games. Teenagers can be very talkative while engrossed in video games! I was happy that I was finally able to see patients.

As I shot the breeze with them, I eventually got to hear their stories. I enjoyed spending time with each person in the Tween Zone. Even so, it was difficult to see and hear what illnesses and struggles—many of them worse than my own situation—these youths had to deal with. Empathizing with and relating to children dealing with hardships was my overall intent during my time at the hospital. Very often, I was filled with gratitude for my circumstances and for the support from loved ones, for my relationship with God, and for the hope my faith gave me to help me persevere and have joy in my life!

Chapter 16

Side Effects

In August of 2019, a few months after I had started in the Tween Zone, I was relaxing at home one evening, when further heart trouble came. My heart had gone into Atrial Fibrillation. I went to the emergency room, and as with almost all ER visits, this took a number of hours. They saw the AFib, but it disappeared while I was there, so I went back home because things had returned to normal, and they hadn't found a cause.

A day or two later, my friend Barbara came to my house to see all my kids (goat kids). As we were talking, I started feeling unaccountably tired. Because I had not seen Barbara for a while—since she had left her job at the hospital—I dealt with the fatigue as best as I could until she left. This was not the greatest choice I've ever made… After she left, I told my dad that we should probably go to the hospital again.

I did not have the worry that I had with my heart issues before. I recall thinking as we drove, *Well, it's okay if this is my time to go.* However, I made it to the ER, and the people there started frantically trying to figure out what may be going on with me. They were about to cut me open for some reason, but then a cardiologist (actually a parent of a former student of my mom's) looked at my record and history and decided that surgery was not necessary.

Instead of cutting me open, the cardiologist put me on a heart medication which lowers the heart rate. I was admitted to the hospital for tests and observation. Thankfully, that doctor figured out what was happening rather than have me go under for some kind of procedure that involved cracking my chest open.

The short summary of what was wrong, was that I had Thyroiditis, thus my thyroid was increasing my heart rate, metabolism, fatigue, and just making me feel awful in different ways; this is because the thyroid regulates metabolism and the hormones. The kicker was that the Thyroiditis had been caused by Amiodarone. This was a very rare side effect for the medicine! Shortly after leaving the hospital and having even more tests, I met with an endocrinologist (thyroid doctor) who talked with me about options to get my thyroid back on track before the final option of removing it.

I didn't want another surgery, so I was all for the pharmaceutical route! The doctor prescribed Prednisone (steroids) which I would take from September to, at the longest, December. The steroids were meant to take all those symptoms away and get my thyroid to regulate everything normally again. I learned that Prednisone is similar to Amiodarone in that both are medicines which work extremely well, but doctors don't like their patients to be on either of them for prolonged periods of time because they can have nasty side effects.

One of the side effects of steroids is that they can cause sleeplessness. For many nights, I woke up in bed at around 3:30. I was wide-awake. That did, however, give me more time and an extra excuse to pray more! After being diagnosed with the thyroid problems, I also had to pee more often whenever I was able to sleep. It was terribly annoying.

I went to the doctor about this and ended up getting a CT scan to make sure my bladder was working well. It turned out I had a bit of blood in my urine, so I ended up going to see a urologist. I have mentioned over and over how I hate catheters, but I couldn't have expected what was to come at that appointment.

There was one test the doctor suggested I do to make absolutely sure that I had no issues with my urinary system, and I nervously agreed. I went to a room and sat on a bed with my legs in stirrups, like they used to have women use during births. Next, to look at my bladder, the doctor pushed a camera right up where the catheter goes. A camera! (I apologize for that mental image!)

I was numbed a little bit, and the procedure lasted only about 30 seconds. But—my gosh! Thankfully everything looked fine, and I had no issues, but I never want another procedure like that in my life! On a side note, while I am glad those types of doctors exist, I don't understand what makes somebody studying to become a doctor decide to specialize in something where they have to look at peoples' undercarriages all day!

Since that August, I routinely had about four different doctor appointments per month. I got tired of having to go visit the doctor. My parents also grew tired of these appointments, and of the driving that came along with them! A number of the visits were blood draws, and several focused on the bladder stuff for a while. However, I also began to learn about the potential side effects of prednisone.

I went to an eye appointment, unrelated to the thyroid issues, and discovered that I had pre-glaucoma—an eye disease that can lead to blindness if left untreated. I learned that this was caused by the steroids. So, in addition to all my medicine, I had to add two different sets of eyedrops, for a total of six drops each day. My brother and I saw the eye doctor quite a bit when we were younger and always hated having to get drops. As an adult, I don't like them any better, but I am much more used to them now!

After more months of numerous doctor visits, November came, and I discovered a symptom of the Thyroiditis that I did not mind. My metabolism was very, very high and I could eat whatever I wanted because I wouldn't gain any weight from it. Sometimes I would even lose weight! I knew that at some point I wouldn't be able to eat without consequence, but for the moment, I enjoyed it! I took a few trips to the grocery store just to look for junk food and other foods which I previously could not eat much of at once without my weight going up. What a great feeling it was to eat without the limitations! I could eat donuts, cookies, cake, candy, fast food; there were so many options. After three weeks of that, the time I wasn't looking forward to came. When I noticed that the numbers on the scale began rising, I stopped the over-indulgence. It was fun while it lasted.

December came, and I looked forward to it because that was when my doctor told me that I would be getting off the steroids. Most of the blood draws were now to check if the steroids had brought my hormone levels back to normal. To my surprise, and especially to my doctor's surprise, while the levels were nearly normal, they still were not where they should have been. The doctor told me that in pretty much all people, the prednisone works after four months, but since it hadn't completely done its job, she would leave me on it for a while longer. Though this was not ideal, things could have been worse.

Chapter 17

The New Year Starts with a Bang

I was able to see in the New Year, 2020, by watching fireworks on the beach in Jaco, Costa Rica. Uncle Ed, Aunt Dee Dee, my parents, and I had gone there after Christmas. We had fun and enjoyed each other's company. My favorite experience in Costa Rica was going to see crocodiles in the river!

About midway through the trip, the top of my foot began to hurt. We took a look and discovered it had become infected. My muscles suddenly involuntarily spasmed and tightened, and it was extremely painful. My parents and I decided to go to a Costa Rican clinic for a diagnosis and figuring out what medicine I could take to heal it. The Costa Rican clinic experience was very different from that in the United States.

We headed to the clinic later that night, and randomly found it despite the lack of signage, it was dimly lit, it was surrounded by a heavy security fence, and it was gated! The appearance was deceiving for a medical center! In the United States clinics, hospitals, and emergency rooms are very well-marked and many times busy, while the clinic I went to in Costa Rica looked nothing like a medical building, and even had most of its interior lights switched off!

After being told what antibiotics I could take for my infected foot, we went to a pharmacy the next day, and by this time my foot was in so much pain that I had stopped wearing my shoes. The circumstances stunk and the antibiotics did not seem to be doing much, but it was still a vacation, so I did not want to let my painful foot ruin the rest of my time in Costa Rica!

By the end of the trip however, I was ready to get back home and get my foot taken care of. After a long trip home, I went to a doctor and was put on some different antibiotics. Additionally, I learned that though primarily caused by the prednisone, the infection was exacerbated by a foot brace I sometimes wore. Prednisone increases the body's chances of getting infections. At this point, I was eager to stop taking steroids!

Around the time I was going through all of this with my foot, I had another blood test to check my hormone levels. I met with my endocrinologist. She told me that, upon seeing the results, she was stumped. My levels had plateaued below where they should be. She had researched the issue, but she was not able to find any articles on a patient whose hormone levels, after being on steroids for five months, hadn't returned to normal levels. Neither had any of the other doctors she conferred with had any experience like this with prednisone. So again, no easy fix for me!

In our discussion, she presented my options. They were to either 1) have my thyroid removed surgically, or 2) basically to stop the steroids, re-start the heart medicine months later, and see if the hormone levels equal out. The second option may not work for sure, and it also was not guaranteed that the heart medicine wouldn't interfere with the thyroid again in the future. I decided on the former. Yes, it was another surgery, but with my thyroid removed, there would be no chance of any further issues with it in the future. So, I scheduled the surgery for the coming spring or summer. That was fine with me; I was sick of all the thyroid stuff.

I had to be on antibiotics for my foot for about six weeks, and after about a week, the infection really began to improve. In February, with my foot beginning to to heal, I made an appointment to consult with a doctor about having new foot braces made. My year was starting off with a bang!

One thing that I had been doing routinely over the number of months since all this trouble began, was checking my blood pressure. The morning of the appointment for new foot braces, I, as usual, checked my blood pressure. When I used the cuff, it showed my blood pressure was fine, but it measured my heart rate at 90 beats per minute. That's higher than usual; my resting pulse should be in the upper 50s to 60s. I thought, *Well that seems high, but I'm going to a doctor today and they always check your blood pressure. It will probably fade away.*

In addition to the higher-than-usual pulse, I also had a lingering cough from some bug I had caught over the previous week. I figured that my high heart rate may have had something to do with whatever I had been fighting off. So, I went to the appointment. The nurse used a blood pressure machine, and it showed my pulse as being in the 90s. The nurse thought this was a bit high, so she tried again. Same thing. She recorded this and then sent me to meet with the doctor.

Throughout that whole morning, even though my heart rate appeared to be higher, I felt normal. I will didn't feel those tired feelings as I do when I feel my AFib kicking in. However, my pulse remained at the same rate as it was earlier, so my dad and I conferred, and he called my cardiologist's office during the appointment.

The cardiologist told my dad that, because my pulse wasn't lowering, I should head to the emergency room when my appointment was finished. Luckily, the hospital was right across the street from the doctor's office, so we didn't have to go too far!

We headed to the hospital, and I calmly went to the emergency room. Eventually, the staff gave me an increase in a medicine dosage which lowered my heart rate. Similar to the previous visit to the ER, the doctors had me start taking the Amiodarone again, as that is a medicine that regulated my heartbeat. I was admitted again, and my heart rate eventually lowered.

Physically, I never felt that anything was wrong! I was just irritated that I had be in a hospital again! I also went in on a Friday, and since hospitals are slower over the weekend, I knew I would be there a few days. This was a boring weekend, being stuck in the hospital in a bed, feeling fine, with not too much to do.

Thankfully, my parents were there, and some family and friends also stopped by and visited. The final Marvel movie had come out and was on the hospital TV's movie list and my dad and I watched it. It didn't make a lot of sense, but we later learned that was because we had watched movie number two, the second part of a two-movie finale without having seen the first.

Soon, Monday came. The cardiologist that my mom knew, whom I had seen on a previous visit, was at the hospital that day and was happy with the progress of my heart over the weekend. My pulse rate was lower, but it still was not maintaining a normal rate after three days. She decided on a procedure called a Cardioversion, where they would attempt to shock my heart back into a regular rhythm; I was a bit nervous about this!

For this procedure, I would not be completely put under. If the cardioversion was successful, I would be able to leave the hospital that same day.

I went to the procedure room and drank some sort of numbing solution. In the procedure they stick a device down the esophagus next to the heart and shock it, like a defibrillator, I surmise. Because of the shock to the heart however, they could only attempt about three times to try to be successful. After dozing off, I woke up a short time later, and thankfully, the first attempt had been a success, and my heart rate was back to normal. I would be able to leave in a couple of hours, around noon! It felt good just to get that over with!

It was so good to be able to go home, but I would still have to drive into town the following evening to have one more follow-up to make sure my heart rate was maintaining. I was simply ready to relax at home, but one more trip wasn't much of a bother.

After getting the all-clear at the appointment that following evening, I got in my van with my dad to head back home while my mom also drove separately from the office. When we were only about three minutes from the doctor's office, I started fiddling with my phone, because it had gotten stuck under my seatbelt. When I started doing this though, I started to feel very badly. A great feeling of the strain and fatigue from the AFib came over me.

Chapter 18

No More Fear

After a few minutes going back and forth with my dad, my breathing labored and I told him, I needed to go to the ER. My dad started driving towards the hospital, which was downtown, and the longer the drive went on, the worse I felt. Breathing became more and more labored, and the amount of air that I could breathe in became less and less. As all this went on, I started to sweat pretty heavily.

My poor dad was speeding his way to the hospital, and I hoped, for his sake, nothing would happen before we got there. We made it to the ER in maybe 20 minutes, probably around 30 miles. Once there, I was rushed into a room and surrounded by people. Things happened very quickly. I was monitored and my heart rate was not going down. At one point my heart rate was 200 BPM! In the moment, that whole episode was very scary.

Nurses scrambled around me, and it was completely unclear as to what would happen. Since my heart rate was so high, they wanted to use a defibrillator to shock my heart into a slower rhythm. A nurse told me, "I hope this isn't your favorite shirt," and proceeded to cut my shirt open on the bed. Then suddenly, just before they prepared to use the defibrillator, my heart rate plummeted to a much lower and more normal level!

That was certainly a God thing; the situation was dire but at the last second, changed for the better. Four years after I had nearly died in an emergency room, the Lord saved my life again! After things calmed down, I was talking with my mom and realized, that *was* one of my favorite shirts!

I was re-admitted into the hospital—just one day after leaving from my recent four-day stay. My parents and I had no idea what was going on, because the procedure I'd had on Monday had already stabilized my heartrate. I thought, *Lord, what is going on?*

The next morning, which was a Wednesday, I saw Dr. Lewkowiez, the electro-physician again (who, four years before, had talked to me about different options for my heart in the future) and this time he told me that an ablation was necessary, and needed to happen soon. He scheduled the procedure for Friday. This was *a lot* to take in; it was Wednesday! Now, not only was the ablation the only option, but it was only two days away, not years!

All I was very unsure about the situation. I knew I needed the procedure… but again, it was risky. Doctors would be working directly on my heart and this without even knowing until once inside if they could even do the procedure! Mainly though, my trepidation stemmed from the fact that it was a heart procedure!

The bigger concern was considering what the doctors told me about being under anesthesia with my physical circumstances. Considering that my heart has already been so affected by Friedreich's, it is a big unknown if my heart has the strength to "wake up" and function on its own after being under anesthesia. This concern was even more worrisome considering the lengthiness of the procedure.

I resolutely told my parents that if I did end up on a ventilator after surgery, I would rather die than be stuck on one of those machines; this was probably my greatest fear. With all this coming up, I had to work on putting all of my trust in God. He was my hope and comfort in this sudden turn of events.

My parents let my siblings know that I was in the hospital again and told them about the upcoming procedure, and they were both able to fly in. Over the next few days, I again had a bustling hospital room. I had so many family members and numerous friends visit with me. Many of my friends I hadn't seen for months! Those days before the ablation were not boring; I was busy conversing with people all the time! I was busy even up to the night before. My brother had decided to spend the night, and when my last visitor, an uncle, left, we attempt this ed to go to sleep.

As I lay in the bed feeling anxious, I began to pray. While I was praying and thinking about the events coming in the morning however, I came to have absolutely no anxiety; the Holy Spirit took over. I undeniably felt the peace God gives which is promised to us in the Bible.

In my prayers I wasn't even focusing on only the events of the next day. I was being encouraged and comforted. I contemplated my life and saw that though I have faced difficulties and suffering, the Lord has always been faithful to help and take care of me. God was reminding and showing me how my life and my faith through my physical struggles have been a witness and have been completely worthwhile. Despite my physical hardships, I haven't got one ounce of bitterness in me; despite all of it and through it all, I have been blessed tremendously! Again, I was reminded that even if I am not healed while on earth, having this very broken body has certainly been worth it if seeds of the Gospel are planted through it.

Regarding my worry about the procedure, one of the things God had me do was to meditate on Jesus and His prayers to the Father in the garden of Gethsemane before his crucifixion. Jesus knew the plan and was aware of what was coming. He knew that he would be sentenced to death. He knew that He would endure mocking, humiliation, and great physical suffering leading up to His death. He knew that he would die in a horrible, painful way—being nailed to a cross and left to slowly suffocate. And He knew that before His death, He would bear the wrong of all of mankind's sins, and that God would turn from Him and reject Him.

I recalled that Jesus knew these things were coming. We are told about this in Matthew 26. Jesus, in his humanity, feared losing His life. In that time of tremendous stress, He prayed, "If it is possible, take this cup from me." Jesus, as a man, really didn't want to go through all of this. "But not my will, but Yours be done." Jesus Christ—the Lord—was terrified of death here on Earth at that time, yet in Jesus' divinity, He trusted God and God's plan, and desired that plan more than His own human desires. And all the while, Jesus could have easily let His worries steer Him away from what the Father had intended for Him. I took great comfort in meditating on all this, knowing that Jesus could relate to me in that moment. I really wanted to be more like Him in that way.

The riskiness of the heart procedure, coupled with the unknowns of anesthesia the next day, made this a high-stakes event. If I were to die, that was fine with me. I wanted *God's will* to be done, rather than mine, even if God's will included death at that time. The fear of death can be tremendous to many.

But in fact, if one's heart is in the right place, death—when it happens in accordance with God's plan—is the best thing that can happen for that individual! The Lord showed me a number of other revelations that night, some of which I cannot even remember now. It was such a glorious night, and I am so thankful for His peace and presence at that moment!

In the morning, I woke up completely refreshed, even though I probably did not get many hours of sleep that night. I concluded that my lack of sleep didn't really matter since I would be ongoing under anesthesia soon anyways. Also of tremendous comfort to me, was that my parents who were praying prior to the procedure, told me that they also were also given peace and assurance.

I went to the preparation room. I had about half-an-hour to visit and pray with my family before heading into the operating room. From the time I had awakened until the time I went under for the surgery, I felt zero worry or anxiety. I was secure with whatever might come to be. The only downside of the day was knowing that I would be getting another catheter!

Although I had come to accept the possibility of death, I was happy to find myself waking up in a hospital bed after the procedure. I came through it! I felt fine but was pretty tired. The only areas I was sore were inside my legs in the crotch region where they had cut incisions to thread the devices through my arteries up to my heart for the ablation. I was very thankful and praised the Lord; it wasn't my time yet!

After the procedure Dr. Lewkowiez summarized how he felt the surgery had gone. He explained that he had spent a lot of time attempting to find and work on one specific area of my heart but had been unable to locate the area. He was very disappointed about this. Even so, he figured on about 60/40 odds of the ablation being successful/unsuccessful. The surgery gave about a 60% chance of getting my heart into a more regular rhythm without the need for heavy heart medication.

These weren't great numbers, but I was pleased. Anything over 50% is positive! So even with those lower-than-hoped-for odds, I wasn't concerned. That night of prayer and peace before surgery had drastically changed my outlook! My faith was matured even more. Thinking back to four years earlier in 2016, when I'd had heart failure and been in the hospital, I could see that my views and thoughts about death had completely changed.

In 2016, I was very afraid. I had always known that, because of my disorder, the day would come—and sooner than later—when I would die. However, I had remained somewhat blissfully ignorant of death. I did not want to think about it or focus on it because it would come whenever it did, and what was the point focusing on it or worrying about it? That view held out and I did not worry about death. But ... when the potential for it came in 2016, I wasn't prepared to face it. That's the human approach; if it's scary, we like to push any thought of it off.

Four years later with the ablation procedure and making it through another life-threatening event, I have no fear of death anymore. I think of death often and have no anxiety; I look forward to it! To be clear: neither my thoughts about death nor my looking forward to it are macabre or morose. My thoughts about dying are not unhealthy. Rather, I want to live every possible day on this earth as fully I can. The thing is, I know what awaits me. I know where I am going when I die. I know how much better things will be in heaven. Most importantly, I know with Whom I will spend eternity! Death will come, and I feel no dread of it. Rather, I look forward to it!

I recently read a book about Dietrich Bonhoeffer, a theologian executed by the Nazis, and some of his words touched my heart. As he was arrested and knew that he would be killed, he told a fellow prisoner, "This is not the end, but for me is the beginning of life."² I know that there is no end for me and that my true life begins when I die. I will close this chapter with some beautiful and powerful words from a sermon that Bonhoeffer gave about death.

> No one has yet believed in God and the kingdom of God, no one has yet heard about the realm of the resurrected, and not been homesick from that hour, waiting and looking forward joyfully to being released from bodily existence.
>
> Whether we are young or old makes no difference. What are twenty or thirty or fifty years in the sight of God? And which of us knows how near he or she may already be to that goal? That life only really begins when it ends here on earth, that all that is here is only the prologue before the of grace that God gives to people who believe in him. Death is mild, death is sweet and gentle; it beckons to us with heavenly power, if only we realize that it is the gateway to our homeland, the tabernacle of joy, the everlasting kingdom of peace.
>
> How do we know that dying is so dreadful? Who knows whether, and our human fear and anguish we are only shivering and show shuddering at the most glorious, heavenly, blessed event in the world? Death is hell and night and cold, if it is not transformed by our faith. But that is just what is so marvelous, that we can transform death.³

Truths I've Experienced

Joy

> Consider it pure joy, my brothers and sisters, whenever you face trials of many kinds, because you know that the testing of your faith produces perseverance.
>
> James 1: 2-3

As I near the end of this book I want to re-emphasize my brokenness. I'm a sinner, and my physical disorder is not the only trouble I have dealt with in the past or continue to deal with presently I have learned many of God's truths throughout my life—especially through my trials. I do my best to live my life according to what I know is right. I strive to apply what I have learned so that my life reflects Christ. I do fall; I don't always live up to who I should be. While I am thankful for how my life has turned out thus far, I certainly am frustrated at times and am not always content. I thank the Lord for His grace and love, and I hope to do whatever I can for Him in my lifetime.

I love the Lord greatly, and while living, I still long for the ability to do many things: I long to walk again, run again, climb again. I would love to drive. I wish I were not limited to locations based on accessibility. I wish I could travel on my own. I wish I could play an instrument again. I wish I could build with my hands in my hobbies again. I would love to be able to pee standing up again—that is a great freedom men have, which I did not fully appreciate until I lost it! I hope to be able to have the ability to walk with a woman holding hands, I hope to be able to dance with a woman again, I hope to have a wife someday. I hope to be able to work a full-time job someday. These are only some of the things I yearn for, yet there are so many more. What will God allow? I do not know.

It can be difficult for me to think about all the things that I deeply desire. Many are things I once could do and have since lost the ability to do. Many, maybe more, are things that I have never done. Even so, the Lord is good. "The LORD gave and the LORD has taken away; may the name of the LORD be praised (Job 1:21)."

While I can compare myself neither to experiencing Job's hardships nor to demonstrating his faithfulness, I had something that was taken. I have lost much that was meaningful to me. I earnestly yearn for all these things. But while I wait, the Lord has both shown me truths and given me a conclusion that I could not have come up with on my own, but rather only in faith.

If I live the rest of my life without God healing me of my physical afflictions, and yet just one person is led to Christ through my trial, testimony, or witness in my circumstances, then a lifetime of physical hardship is completely worth it! To God be the glory!

In dealing with my physical trial, I have come to greatly appreciate and understand more and more the exhortation given to believers in James 1:2-3 to meet trials with joy.

At face value and without any context, this seems like a ludicrous declaration! And in context, it seems even worse! James was writing to Jewish Christians who were enduring much persecution. Trial and joy don't seem to go together; and—usually—they don't! But, as you have read, I have great joy in my trial! I have that future hope and knowledge that what I am living with is not permanent. James 1:4 continues to describe why perseverance in life is so important. "Let perseverance finish its work so that you may be mature and complete, not lacking anything." The perseverance (patience, endurance, steadfastness) which was developed in a time of trial, or testing, works to make faith complete! It is in times of trial when a person can grow closest to God and become more mature as a Christian.

I rejoice in trials because I know that God does much good—both for me and for others—through them. Though I do not suffer directly for Christ's name, I am privileged to live with my adversity, doing what I can to glorify Him and to be a witness and a servant to others in their own adversity. For the Christian, times of tribulation are opportunities for others to see God in and through them. It would not make sense to an unbeliever, but being in a relationship with Jesus is where the joys and blessings from trials can be found.

Chapter 19

Conclusion

What I've written is a general summary of my life up to this point. As I wrote at the beginning, I'm not very old—only in my younger 30s. And as you can see, I have not really accomplished terribly much of significance thus far in my lifetime. I am still living with Friedreich's Ataxia daily. My legs are weak but useful, and the nerves in my hands and fingers have continued to weaken. Additionally, my fingers have curled, and my dexterity is much more limited. When I hear a recording of myself, I cringe and wish I was clearer and more elegant while speaking. There are other different issues that bother me in my insecurity, but I try not to focus on these. I'm single, and there are times when I desire a wife someday. That being said and acknowledged, I have gotten to a point where I am continuing to learn to be content with being single and don't foresee that type of relationship in my life, for a number of reasons. A wife may still be a blessing in the future, but if not, that just simply isn't in God's plan for me! I hope to be able to get a job that will allow me to be able to provide. For multiple reasons, I'm physically not able to have a job where I work full-time every week. This is another thing I am relying on God for in my future: provision. As noted before, I have many desires, but my greatest desire is to serve the Lord, who has blessed me greatly! I pray for more opportunities to share my faith and my testimony, and for Christ to work through me.

In the danger that any of what you read has elevated my status in your mind, or in the possibility that I have made myself sound righteous, allow me to humble myself. I am simply a normal guy. My life isn't spectacular, and there are people with faith and/or stories that are much more inspirational than my own. In being normal, I excel at sinning. My thoughts aren't always pure, my tongue isn't always under control, nor are my words always to God's glory. As with most men, lust is a big struggle. I do not always treat people the way they should be treated. I certainly don't trust God as much as I should. I sometimes harbor anger, and in my sin, I am hypocritical of many of the teachings of the Bible according to which I strive to live. I am not going to share all my sins in detail, but rest assured, there are, and have been, many. I am no special or holy man; I am simply a sinner saved by grace doing my best to serve the Lord and to improve my life by striving to follow Jesus' teachings. The Bible makes it clear that no person is worth more or less than another, and I don't view myself at either end.

The common theme in this book and in my life has been my physical trial and growing in it and through it. My true life's theme, however, has nothing to do with that. My physical trial has been a blessing in so many parts of my life, as God has shown Himself faithful time and time again when I have needed strength and hope. But none of this ultimately matters, not without a purpose. The reason that I am a Christian, and the reason that I am what I am, has nothing to do with my earthly experiences and seeing God in them. The reason has to do with something which I did not personally witness, but has tremendously benefited me.

Specifically, the reason is that because of Jesus' unfathomable love for me and for you—for all mankind, He came to this earth, was born to a virgin as both God and man. He lived and taught how people should live their lives, honoring their Creator. The leadership of the established religion schemed against Him, and he was unjustly sentenced to crucifixion.

Prior to being nailed to a cross, because of His love for us, Jesus was mocked, flogged, and given a crown of thorns. Because of His love for us, Jesus was forced to carry His cross to the execution site, while being subjected to more humiliation along the way. Because of His love for us, God allowed His Son to be nailed to the cross. Because of His love for us, the cross was erected, and Jesus suffered agonizing emotional, spiritual, physical pain for hours until He died, taking the wrath of God upon Himself for humanity's sinfulness. Upon Jesus' death the curtain—which symbolized the separation between humanity and God—was torn. And because of Jesus' love for us, He was resurrected from death three days later. In His victory over death (Christ's death and resurrection), Jesus brought humanity the path to salvation not only from Hell, but from ourselves, and from our sins, sorrows, and sicknesses.

This path is open to all who choose to believe. More amazingly, the way to salvation is based neither on works nor on reliance on one's own actions. Salvation and grace, the undeserved forgiveness of our wrongs, are given freely if one simply acknowledges that Jesus Christ is Savior and Lord.

This is what drives my life. Again, I'm a Christian not because of God's help given to me in my struggles with my body; I'm a Christian, first and foremost, because of Jesus' unfathomable love and sacrifice for me. Not only do I have a valuable relationship with the Lord in this life, but I also have the hope of living in eternal perfection with Him when I die.

This, the Gospel, is the foundation of my life. From the Gospel, I work to develop my character and attitude. Certainly, I am not perfect, but I do the best job I can to live by the Bible's teachings.

I cannot put into words how thankful and grateful I am that Jesus sacrificed Himself for me, offering me salvation! It is something I certainly cannot repay! Yet as a Christian living from gratitude, I can love and serve others according to His commands, and I want to be a witness sharing the Gospel to those in need of it. In writing this book, my hopes and prayers are that my testimony will serve as both a witness and as an encouragement to you, and that you will see the need for Jesus in your life!

Deo Gloria—To God Be the Glory!

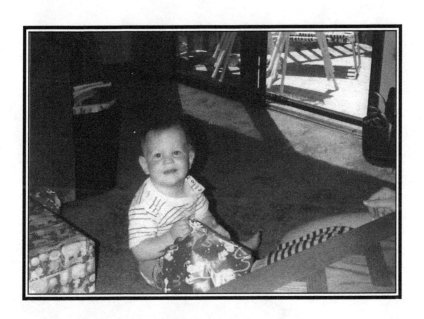

David as a baby.

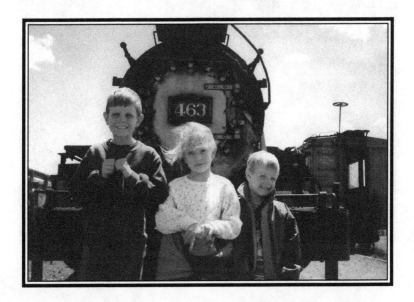

David, Jeanelle, and Daniel at the Cumbres and Toltec RR.

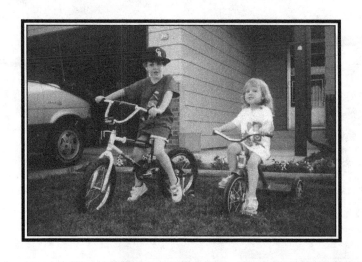

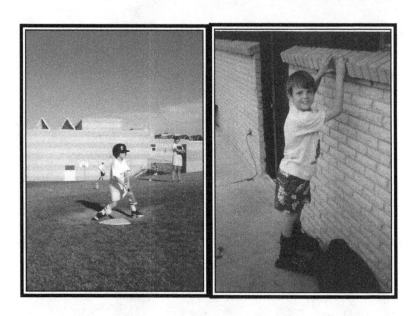

David engaging in childhood activities.

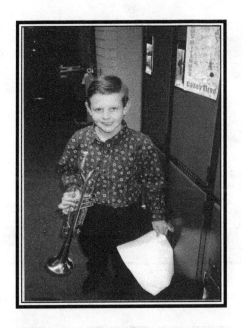

David a few months before diagnosis.

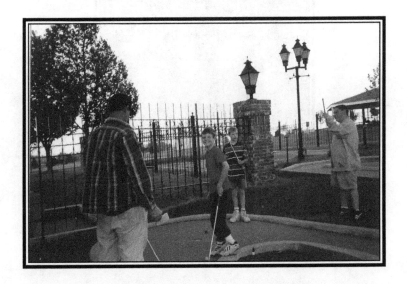

A few months after diagnosis.

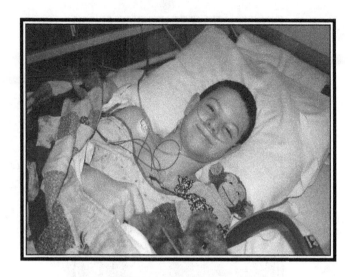

David recovering in the hospital after the first spinal fusion surgery.

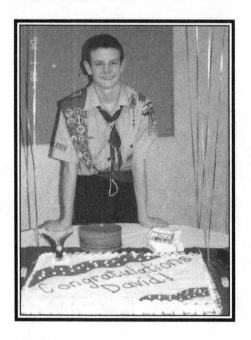

Having received the Eagle Scout award.

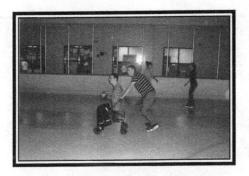

Aaron and David playing around on an ice rink at an after prom.

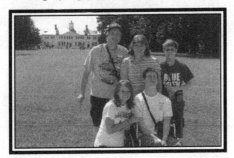

On a family vacation in high school. (We used a wheelchair rather than the walker on trips because of the long distances).

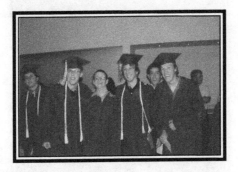

High school friends, Geoff "IB" Scott, Aaron, me, Tyler, Matt Klements, Matt Kok.

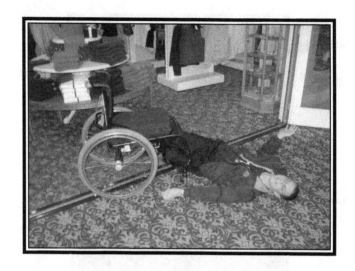

On the floor at the Broadmoor.

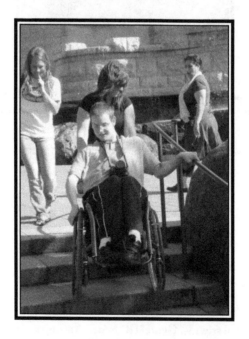

going down a set of stairs in Washington DC.

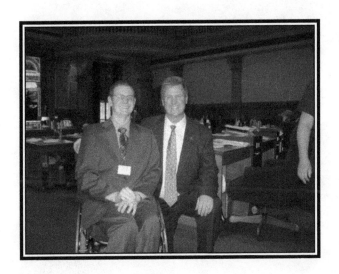

Senator Scott Renfroe and I.

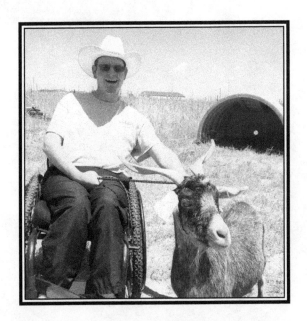

David and Ramona.

Afterword

As I write this book, it is the last half of 2021. My heart ablation was performed over a year-and-a-half ago, and I am happy to say that with only a 60% chance of success, the procedure has proven to have been successful! For most of 2021 I have not been taking Amiodarone. Though I still take heart medications, no medication to help control my heart rhythm is needed at this point! In this blessing, I've been freed from taking a medicine that creates harsh side effects.

From what I have been told, the ablation was done pretty much for the purpose of giving me some more years of life. It is temporary, and I don't know how long it will last before I will have to start on the Amiodarone again. There will also come a time to consider future options which are becoming more limited. At this point, however, since the ablation, my heart has been healthy and feeling great! I've made a habit each day of thanking God for yet another day of life with such good health. I know it is very easy to take that for granted, so I must remember to rejoice in it!

Since my ablation, I have had one other surgery. With all the thyroid problems I had, my doctor wanted my thyroid removed in 2020. Everything with my heart was unexpected, but even after I left the hospital in February, the thyroidectomy was still supposed to take place that spring or summer. I was somewhat unsure of how all of this would work out, because in March, all of the COVID stuff began. Everything was shutting down or getting restricted, so I didn't even know if my thyroid procedure would happen.

At that time, I was very thankful that everything with my heart happened in February, because I had been able to see so many people before common activities ground to a halt. Though many people experienced the cancellation of their scheduled medical procedures during 2020, mine must have been necessary enough to squeak through. I was scheduled for a thyroidectomy in June. After my ablation and what the Lord revealed to me, I had come to the point in which I had zero worries about this surgery. I also knew that everything had gone well with the anesthesia before, so that wouldn't be a problem.

The only anxiety I had was in the requirement I get a COVID test the weekend before the surgery. I know that the test is not really a big deal, but I had heard about it, and I knew that having a stick jammed up my nose would be very uncomfortable! I went to have my test done and I received some of God's mercy that day. They stuck the thing up my nose a bit and then towards my throat some. This was contrary to what I'd heard, so I asked if the procedure had changed. The nurse told me that very recently they had changed to this method of testing as it is more accurate. I don't know if the tests remained that way or if they reverted to the "brain surgery" method—as I've heard it called. But whatever it was, God gave me grace in that!

The whole experience leading up to my thyroid surgery was very foreign to me. Usually when I know a surgery is coming up, I have some anxiety! In the days before, it seemed like I was just going to run an errand. It was so weird. In reality, the surgeon was going to cut into the lower part of my neck and remove my thyroid—a necessary body part— and hopefully not nick anything important like the vocal cords or little things called parathyroids that surround the thyroid (if these are affected in surgery, larger issues can be created regarding calcium levels and metabolism). Even this, though, did not make me anxious. At the hospital, as I was prepped for surgery, wheeled into the operating room, and while I was waiting in the operating room, I felt no fear. I had been prepared and knew that God's will would be done, and even if that meant something more would happen to me, I knew that it was nothing to fear!

I woke up, and felt the usual grogginess and fatigue after surgery, but was delighted that I did not wake up with a catheter! (This is the last time I will mention catheters!) That surgery was short enough that there was no need for one, thank goodness! I had to stay overnight just to make sure everything was good, but then I got to go home.

My time in the hospital was unbelievable. I figured that my neck would be sore where the incision was, but I had no pain! I was tired from the surgery, but never even took a nap that afternoon after surgery. Except for the one painkiller the nurse gave me right after surgery, I didn't take any more medication.

The surgery and hospital experiences were incredibly easy, and it felt like I had gone in for something minor! Even over the following months of recovery—except for the one time in the hospital—I never took any pain medicine, and I had no issues with stamina, with pain, with side effects, with anything. It was so dang easy! I wondered, *Lord, thank you so much, but I'm not sure why you made this so easy!*

So, all went successfully and now I am just required to take synthetic hormone pills every day because I can't produce these naturally anymore! Since the ablation and the thyroidectomy,

I am doing very well physically! Again, I don't know how long this will last, but I'm trusting in my Lord's will each day.

With all the chaos from the politics and from the restrictions with COVID, the opportunity to get back to the hospital and a volunteer has not yet worked out. But I am seeking opportunities within my church and other groups. Again, my faith, which is becoming more and more mature, gives me confidence in this pandemic situation. So many people are terrified of contracting the virus, but this has to with what or who's one's trust and hope is in. Simply put, I don't want to get sick, but if I do get the virus and die from it, there is not much I can do about it. And if I do die, I have no fear of it!

References

[1] Strong, Strong's Concordance 232.

[2] Metaxas, Bonhoeffer, 528

[3] Metaxas, Bonhoeffer, 530-531

Bibliography

Metaxas, Eric. *Bonhoeffer: Pastor, Martyr, Prophet, Spy.* Nashville: Thomas Nelson Publishers, 2010.

Strong, James. *The New Strong's Expanded Exhaustive Concordance of the Bible.* Nashville: Thomas Nelson Publishers, 2010.